BEATING ANXIETY & DEPRESSION
14 Natural Secrets to a Happier Life

Dr. Joseph Jacobs, DPT, ACN

First Edition, May 2025
Published by ASTR Institute
614 E HWY 50 #169, Clermont, FL 34711

ASTR

ASTRinstitute.com

Disclaimer

This book, authored by Dr. Joseph Jacobs and published by the ASTR Institute, is intended for informational purposes only and presents medical research findings. It is not a substitute for professional medical advice, diagnosis, or treatment. Dr. Joseph Jacobs, the ASTR Institute, and its affiliates do not endorse or assume responsibility for any specific medical treatments or procedures discussed in this book. We strongly advise readers to consult with their healthcare providers regarding the applicability of any aspects of the content to their own health and well-being.

The statements contained herein have not been evaluated by the Food and Drug Administration. The products mentioned are not designed to diagnose, cure, treat, or prevent any disease. Individual results may vary, and we cannot guarantee that you will achieve the same outcomes as those detailed in our case studies, testimonials, and treatment videos. Success varies per individual, and one person's results do not guarantee similar outcomes for another.
If you have medical concerns, consult with your healthcare provider, physician, or another qualified medical professional. Dr. Joseph Jacobs, the ASTR Institute, and their associated organizations and individuals disclaim any liability for actions, services, or products acquired through this book, our videos, website, or any of our media channels.

Table of Contents

Online Resources

How to Access Online Resources

Throughout this book, you'll find barcodes that link to additional online resources. Here's how to use them:

1. Open the camera app on your smartphone.
2. Point the camera at the barcode.
3. A notification will appear with a link. Tap the notification to open the link in your browser.

Triumph Over Trials: My Journey from Disability to Victory

Triumph Over Trials

After my second cancer treatment, I was suffering from chronic fatigue, migraines, muscle and joint pain. I reached out to at least seven doctors, but I could not find relief. Unfortunately, they had two responses. First, they said my blood labs looked normal. I learned from my studies in nutrition that this happened because they did not order the correct labs to figure out the root cause of my issues. The second response was that I was a hopeless case. This made me realize that if I wanted to overcome my disability, I had to look for a solution on my own. It was a difficult time in my life. Due to my pain and fatigue, it used to take me 10 minutes just to walk from the living room to the bathroom, about 20 feet away. I was very depressed and angry because, at 30 years old, I was facing numerous health issues and had a poor quality of life without any answers.

I spent countless hours and years studying nutrition, psychology, behavioral modification, anatomy, physiology, ergonomics, and other medical topics in hopes of finding an answer. At the same time, I was frustrated that the techniques I learned in medical school only provided short-term results with no lasting relief. I tried what I learned in school, such as stretching, exercises, electrical stimulation, various massage techniques, manual therapy, joint mobilization, and myofascial release, but nothing provided long-term results. So, I started to look at medical studies to guide me through this process. After reviewing over 16,000 medical research papers with assistance from medical students, I was shocked and disappointed by the results. Based on these studies, the following treatments either provided no pain reduction or only short-term pain reduction:

- NSAIDs
- Opioids
- Cortisone shots
- Exercises
- Stretching
- Massage
- Joint mobilization or manipulation
- Acupuncture
- Dry needling
- Instrument-assisted soft tissue mobilization

I have dedicated my life to researching all current traditional medical approaches to treating pain. I've found that the majority of these approaches primarily focus on relieving symptoms rather than addressing the root cause of the pain. The techniques I learned in school, still used in today's modern medical world, have their origins in ancient healing practices such as manipulation, massage, stretching, and exercise. These methods were used by the Romans, Greeks, and Egyptians to increase flexibility, strengthen muscles, and alleviate pain. Today's medicine has added treatments like cold, heat, electrical stimulation, and joint adjustment to this list. However, overwhelming evidence from published medical studies shows no promising long-term relief from any of these methods.

For instance, one systematic review conducted by the University of Ottawa, Canada, which reviewed 270 research studies, concluded that the benefits of massage, acupuncture, and spine adjustment treatments were mostly evident immediately or shortly after treatment, then faded over time. With compelling data like this, it is perplexing how we continue to treat patients with modalities that do not effectively address their long-term needs. Instead of focusing so much on the body's symptoms, we need to start questioning why these symptoms are present in the first place and why they keep returning.

This question guided me through an intense investigative research process over five years. From this research, I concluded that there are seven aspects of chronic pain that, when treated simultaneously, can lead to long-term pain relief. In my book, **Pain No More**, I outline seven key elements that must be addressed simultaneously to effectively relieve chronic pain. I also found that the BioPsychosocial model is an effective treatment approach for long-term pain reduction. So, I studied the BioPsychosocial model in depth and realized that my medical education was lacking in nutrition knowledge. I spent thousands of hours reading and studying nutrition and bought any book that I felt could help me understand the body better.

During this time, my wife had chronic jaw pain due to stress at work. I tried everything I learned from school on her, but nothing provided long-term pain relief. One day she woke up with lockjaw, unable to speak or open her mouth. She asked me to try anything. I told her that I had tried everything I knew, but nothing worked. So, I reached inside her mouth and experimented with several maneuvers. After a few minutes, she was able to open her mouth and was pain-free. I was dumbfounded and had no idea what had just happened. It took me several days to understand the physiology of the maneuvers I had performed. I then started experimenting with the same concept, applying it to the whole body to relieve both my pain and my patients' pain.

After several months of using my hands to implement the new maneuvers I had come up with, I realized I could not do that long-term. My hands were very sore, and I suffered from pain every night. I told my wife that this was not sustainable because I was in so much pain from using my hands. While patients were getting relief, I was suffering. My wife suggested that I use tools instead of my hands. So, I went to a hardware store and bought rubber, plastic, and metal to cut and design tools and devices to replace my hand maneuvers. Thankfully, this provided even faster results for my patients without me feeling soreness from working on them.

I was able to overcome my chronic fatigue and migraines by running comprehensive lab tests. These tests revealed several vitamin, mineral, and hormonal imbalances. Additionally, I overcame my chronic joint and muscle pain through the biopsychosocial (BPS) model and the tools and devices I invented. I also reinvented the biopsychosocial model to be implemented by a single healthcare provider and called it ASTR treatment.

My journey toward developing the ASTR diet was driven by personal challenges and professional insights. I experienced significant frustration with various diets that often left me feeling fatigued and unsatisfied. Through an extensive review of research studies, I also uncovered potential health risks associated with extreme dietary approaches. These experiences inspired me to create the ASTR Diet as a healthier, evidence-based alternative, which I share in my book *Eat to Heal*.

For years, I suffered from debilitating **depression and PTSD**, searching for lasting relief beyond temporary fixes. My journey as both a patient and a healthcare provider led me to dedicate 15 years to researching, studying, and testing effective solutions. Through this process, I developed a comprehensive approach that transformed my own health and has helped countless patients overcome **chronic depression and PTSD**. In this book, I share these evidence-based strategies, solutions that I have refined through experience and clinical practice. My hope is that this book serves as a practical guide to empower you on your path to recovery, providing the tools and knowledge needed to reclaim a **happier, healthier life**.

The Roadmap to Healing

The Roadmap to Healing: A Comprehensive Approach to Beating Anxiety and Depression

Depression and anxiety are among the most complex and misunderstood conditions, often presenting as more than just low mood or excessive worry. They are systemic issues influenced by multiple underlying factors that vary from person to person. Through 15 years of research, clinical practice, and personal experience, I have found that depression and anxiety are rarely triggered by a single cause. Instead, they result from a combination of factors such as chronic stress, hormonal imbalances, inflammatory foods, environmental toxins, gut health disruptions, deficiencies in essential vitamins and minerals, and unresolved trauma. Many individuals struggling with depression and anxiety have at least seven to ten contributing triggers, making an individualized and holistic approach to treatment essential for lasting relief.

In this chapter, I introduce a structured roadmap to healing, 14 natural secrets to lasting relief designed to address the root causes of depression and anxiety rather than just suppressing symptoms. These elements are interconnected, and for the best results, it is crucial to implement all 14. Each component plays a key role in restoring balance to the body, reducing inflammation, supporting brain health, and regulating the nervous system. When one or more of these factors are overlooked, depression and anxiety often persist or return, which is why a comprehensive approach is necessary.

By following this roadmap, you are not just managing depression and anxiety; you are taking control of your health and actively working toward healing at its source. This method is not about quick fixes or temporary relief; it's about equipping your body and mind with the tools they need to heal naturally and sustainably. With dedication and consistency, you can break free from chronic depression and anxiety and regain your quality of life, just as I did and as my patients have done.

This book serves as a practical roadmap, guiding you through 14 essential secrets that can help you break free from depression naturally. These principles have transformed my own life and the lives of countless patients. Each chapter introduces a key area that plays a significant role in mental and emotional recovery, providing you with scientific insights, practical strategies, and step-by-step guidance to help you reclaim control over your mind and body.

1. Food and Depression

The journey to emotional healing begins on your plate. This chapter explores the powerful connection between what you eat and how you feel, highlighting how inflammatory foods, processed sugars, and chemical-laden meals can disrupt brain chemistry and intensify depressive symptoms. Nourishing the brain with anti-inflammatory, whole foods is a crucial first step toward stabilizing mood and energy. Without addressing food as a foundational element, other interventions may fall short in reversing depression.

2. Vitamins, Minerals and Hormones Imbalance

Your body cannot function optimally, especially emotionally, without essential nutrients and balanced hormones. This chapter uncovers how deficiencies in vitamins like B12, D3, folate, magnesium, and imbalances in thyroid, cortisol, or sex hormones can trigger or worsen depressive states. Correction of these biochemical imbalances is vital. If left untreated, they can block recovery, even when therapy or medication is used.

3. Drug-Induced Depression

Not all depression is rooted in life circumstances; some is chemically induced. This chapter reveals how certain prescription medications, such as hormonal birth control, corticosteroids, and even antidepressants, can paradoxically contribute to depressive symptoms. Understanding which substances may be influencing your mood helps reclaim control over your emotional state.

4. Brain Glitches: Your Thoughts Are Not You

Although thoughts may be persistent, loud, and convincing, they are not necessarily facts. In this chapter, we explore how to develop awareness that negative thoughts are not reflections of your identity or truth. By learning to observe rather than absorb, you can begin to free yourself from mental loops that fuel depression.

5. Distance Yourself & Zoom Out

When emotions are intense, it's easy to lose perspective. This chapter teaches the practice of cognitive defusion. It shows you how to create space between yourself and your thoughts. By "zooming out," you become less reactive and more resilient. You shift from being inside the storm to observing it calmly from the outside.

6. Trauma Closure: BioPsycho Therapy (BPT)

BPT is a breakthrough trauma-informed approach that addresses the physiological and emotional roots of depression. By combining magnetic stimulation and trauma exposure techniques, BPT works to release stored trauma from the nervous system. This chapter explains that bringing unresolved pain into treatment, rather than avoiding it, is essential for lasting healing. Trauma closure is a crucial step in the healing process, as unresolved trauma can lead to chronic pain, emotional distress, and long-term health issues. BioPsycho Therapy (BPT) is a highly effective tool for achieving trauma closure because it addresses both the psychological and physical aspects of trauma.

7. The Illusion of Control

Clinging to control can create tension, fear, and frustration. This chapter explores how the desire to control people, outcomes, or the future can lead to chronic stress and hopelessness. Letting go of what you cannot control is liberating and opens the door to acceptance and emotional peace.

8. Change is the Only Constant

Depression often stems from resistance to change, whether it's loss, aging, or uncertainty. This chapter encourages embracing change as a natural part of life. By shifting your mindset, change becomes less threatening and more empowering, supporting emotional flexibility and healing.

9. Forgiveness

The Roadmap to Healing

Unforgiveness creates a prison within. Holding on to resentment or guilt can fuel chronic emotional pain. This chapter gently guides you through the process of releasing others and yourself from blame, opening the path to peace, clarity, and emotional freedom.

10. Limit Screen Time

Screens dominate modern life, but their overuse is linked to anxiety, sleep disturbances, and depression. This chapter examines the neuroscience behind digital overstimulation and offers strategies to reduce screen time, helping to restore mental clarity and emotional regulation.

11. Declutter Your Home

Your environment reflects and influences your internal state. A cluttered, chaotic home can increase anxiety and depressive feelings. This chapter explores how creating physical space supports mental space and invites calm and focus into your life.

12. Simplify Your Life

Complexity drains energy. This chapter encourages reevaluating commitments, routines, and expectations to identify what truly matters. Simplifying your life can free up mental bandwidth and reduce the burden that contributes to depressive overwhelm.

13. Mindfulness and Meditation

Being present is healing. In this chapter, we explore how mindfulness and meditation help rewire the brain, reduce stress, and increase emotional awareness. Even a few minutes a day can create powerful changes in mood and perception.

14. Behavior Modification

Changing behavior is the final piece of the puzzle. This chapter explains how

10

small, consistent behavioral shifts such as improving sleep hygiene, increasing movement, and setting goals can create momentum toward emotional stability. By transforming habits, you reshape your emotional baseline.

While each of these 14 elements offers value on its own, true healing occurs when they work together. **The foundation of recovery lies in addressing core physiological and emotional imbalances, such as vitamin and mineral deficiencies, hormonal disruptions, inflammatory food intake, and unresolved trauma.** <u>Without resolving these underlying issues, progress may be limited or temporary</u>. These first pillars build the structure, and the remaining elements complete it, offering the long-term support needed for full and lasting recovery from depression.

Your Journey Begins Now

Healing is not about quick fixes. It's about making small, consistent changes that restore balance to your mind and body. Each of these 14 secrets plays a crucial role in your recovery journey. By addressing inflammation, mindset, environment, and behavior patterns, you can create a life free from depression, stress, and emotional instability.

This book is your guide to lasting mental wellness. I've been where you are, and I know healing is possible. Now, it's time to take the first step. One that leads to clarity, freedom, and lasting well-being.

Understanding Anxiety & Depression

Depression: A Symptom, Not a Disease

Depression is not a standalone disease but rather a symptom associated with a multitude of medical conditions, ranging from neurological disorders to metabolic and inflammatory diseases. Research supports the notion that depression often arises as a consequence of underlying physiological dysfunctions rather than being an independent disorder. For instance, a study by Dantzer et al. (2008) highlights that chronic inflammation plays a significant role in the development of depressive symptoms. The researchers found that patients with elevated levels of pro-inflammatory cytokines, such as interleukin-6 (IL-6) and tumor necrosis factor-alpha (TNF-α), exhibited symptoms of depression, suggesting that inflammation-driven biological changes contribute to mood disturbances rather than an intrinsic psychiatric disorder.

Similarly, metabolic diseases such as diabetes and hypothyroidism frequently present with depressive symptoms, further reinforcing the idea that depression is a secondary manifestation rather than a disease itself. A longitudinal study by Katon et al. (2010) found that individuals with diabetes were twice as likely to develop depressive symptoms compared to non-diabetic individuals. The study emphasized that dysregulated glucose metabolism, insulin resistance, and systemic inflammation contribute to mood disturbances, indicating that treating the metabolic dysfunction could alleviate depressive symptoms. Likewise, hypothyroidism, a condition characterized by reduced thyroid hormone production, is well-documented to cause depressive symptoms due to hormonal imbalances affecting neurotransmitter activity (Hage & Azar, 2012). When hypothyroidism is properly treated with thyroid hormone replacement, depressive symptoms often resolve, further suggesting that depression in such cases is a symptom rather than a primary disease.

Furthermore, neurodegenerative diseases like Parkinson's and Alzheimer's disease frequently present with depression as an early symptom, further challenging the classification of depression as a disease in itself. Research by Aarsland et al. (2011) indicates that nearly 50% of patients with Parkinson's disease experience depressive symptoms, which are largely attributed to neurochemical alterations, particularly in dopamine and serotonin pathways. Similarly, in Alzheimer's disease, depression often precedes cognitive decline, with evidence suggesting that amyloid-beta accumulation and neuroinflammation contribute to mood disturbances (Ownby et al., 2006). These findings reinforce the argument that depression arises as a symptom of underlying pathophysiological changes rather than an independent psychiatric disorder.

Given the substantial evidence linking depression to various medical conditions, it is critical to shift the paradigm from treating it as a distinct disease to addressing its root causes. Studies show that interventions targeting inflammation, metabolic health, and neurochemical imbalances are more effective in managing depressive symptoms than conventional antidepressant treatments alone (Miller & Raison, 2016). Thus, recognizing depression as a symptom rather than a disease could lead to more effective, individualized treatment approaches that focus on the underlying pathology rather than merely suppressing symptoms.

Rethinking Depression: Why Neurotransmitter Imbalance Is Not the Root Cause

The widely held belief that depression is primarily caused by a chemical imbalance, specifically a deficiency in neurotransmitters like serotonin or dopamine, has come under increasing scientific scrutiny. While neurotransmitters do play a role in mood regulation, recent research indicates that this theory is overly simplistic and potentially misleading. A comprehensive review published in *Molecular Psychiatry* by Moncrieff et al. (2022) evaluated decades of research and concluded that there is "no consistent evidence" supporting the idea that low serotonin levels are the direct cause of depression. This challenges the foundation of the "chemical imbalance" hypothesis that has long influenced the use of antidepressant medications such as selective serotonin reuptake inhibitors (SSRIs).

One critical oversight in this theory is the assumption that the body naturally produces sufficient neurotransmitters independent of nutritional status. However, **the body cannot synthesize these neurotransmitters without essential precursors, including vitamins and minerals** such as vitamin B6, B12, folate, magnesium, and zinc. These micronutrients are required for the enzymatic reactions that convert amino acids into neurotransmitters like serotonin and dopamine. For example, vitamin B6 is a cofactor in the conversion of tryptophan to serotonin, while magnesium is essential for dopamine synthesis. A deficiency in these nutrients impairs the body's ability to produce and regulate neurotransmitters, potentially leading to symptoms of depression (Sathyanarayana Rao et al., 2008; Kaplan et al., 2007).

The problem with pharmaceutical interventions such as SSRIs or dopamine agonists is that they do not address these underlying nutrient deficiencies. Instead, they artificially manipulate neurotransmitter levels by inhibiting reuptake or increasing release, which may deplete the body's limited reserves over time.

Since the foundational nutrient imbalance remains uncorrected, the effectiveness of these medications tends to diminish, leading to tolerance, dependency, and in some cases, worsening depression and suicidal ideation (Hengartner, 2017). In essence, the medication may provide short-term symptom relief while exacerbating long-term imbalances due to the body's inability to replenish neurotransmitter stores without sufficient nutritional support.

Therefore, **addressing vitamin and mineral deficiencies is essential for restoring the body's natural ability to produce and regulate neurotransmitters.** Nutritional psychiatry, an emerging field, emphasizes this approach and is increasingly supported by studies showing significant improvements in mood disorders through targeted nutritional interventions (Sarris et al., 2015). Ultimately, a more holistic and evidence-based approach to treating depression should consider nutritional status as a core factor, rather than relying solely on pharmaceutical modulation of neurotransmitters.

Understanding Anxiety

What Is Anxiety?

Anxiety is a complex emotional and physiological response that arises when an individual perceives a threat, whether real or imagined. While anxiety is a normal part of life, serving as a survival mechanism that prepares the body to face danger, it becomes problematic when it is chronic, excessive, or disproportionate to the situation. According to the American Psychiatric Association (2022), anxiety disorders are the most prevalent class of mental disorders in the United States, affecting nearly 30% of adults at some point in their lives.

How Anxiety Affects the Nervous System

At the neurological level, anxiety involves key brain structures and systems. The **amygdala**, a central component of the brain's fear circuitry, plays a pivotal role by detecting threats and triggering a cascade of responses. Once activated, the amygdala signals the hypothalamus to engage the hypothalamic-pituitary-adrenal (HPA) axis, which releases stress hormones like cortisol and adrenaline (Shin & Liberzon, 2010). These hormones initiate the "fight or flight" response, increasing heart rate, respiration, and muscle tension to prepare the body for immediate action. Simultaneously, the sympathetic branch of the autonomic nervous system becomes dominant, while the prefrontal cortex, responsible for rational thinking, becomes less active under stress, leading to impaired decision-making and heightened emotional reactivity (Arnsten, 2009).

Physical Effects of Anxiety on the Body

Chronic anxiety can have a profound impact on the body. Persistent activation of the stress response system may lead to cardiovascular strain, elevated blood pressure, gastrointestinal disturbances such as nausea and irritable bowel syndrome, respiratory problems like hyperventilation, and compromised immune function due to prolonged cortisol exposure (McEwen, 2007; Glaser & Kiecolt-Glaser, 2005). These physical manifestations often reinforce the psychological symptoms of anxiety, creating a vicious cycle that affects overall health and well-being.

Types of Anxiety Disorders

The Diagnostic and Statistical Manual of Mental Disorders, Fifth Edition (DSM-5) outlines several distinct types of anxiety disorders, each with specific characteristics. Below are the major categories:

1. Generalized Anxiety Disorder (GAD)

GAD is characterized by persistent and excessive worry about various aspects of daily life such as work, health, finances, or family. This worry is difficult to control and lasts for at least six months. Symptoms often include restlessness, fatigue, irritability, muscle tension, and sleep disturbances (American Psychiatric Association, 2022).

2. Panic Disorder

Panic disorder involves recurrent and unexpected panic attacks, sudden surges of intense fear or discomfort that reach a peak within minutes. These episodes are often accompanied by physical symptoms such as chest pain, heart palpitations, shortness of breath, dizziness, and fear of losing control or dying. Individuals may also develop anticipatory anxiety, where they fear having another attack (Roy-Byrne, Craske, & Stein, 2006).

3. Social Anxiety Disorder (Social Phobia)

Social anxiety disorder is marked by a persistent fear of being watched, judged, or humiliated in social or performance situations. This can severely interfere with daily functioning, leading individuals to avoid speaking in public, eating in front of others, or attending social events. Physical symptoms may include blushing, trembling, or nausea (Stein & Stein, 2008).

4. Specific Phobias

Specific phobias involve an intense, irrational fear of a specific object or situation, such as heights, animals, flying, or needles. Exposure to the feared stimulus almost always triggers immediate anxiety, which can lead to avoidance behaviors that disrupt daily life. Unlike general anxiety, the fear in phobias is highly focused and disproportionate to the actual danger.

5. Separation Anxiety Disorder

Though commonly diagnosed in children, separation anxiety disorder can also occur in adults. It involves excessive fear or anxiety about being separated from attachment figures such as a parent, spouse, or child. Symptoms may include nightmares, physical complaints, or intense worry about harm coming to loved ones during periods of separation (American Psychiatric Association, 2022).

6. Agoraphobia

Agoraphobia is the fear of being in situations where escape might be difficult or help might not be available in the event of a panic attack or other distressing symptoms. This can include being in crowds, on public transportation, or outside of the home alone. In severe cases, individuals may become housebound.

Each anxiety disorder shares core features of fear and avoidance, but the triggers, manifestations, and patterns of behavior vary significantly.

Causes and Contributing Factors

The causes of anxiety disorders are multifactorial. Genetics play a significant role, with heritability estimates ranging between 30% and 50% depending on the specific disorder (Hettema, Neale, & Kendler, 2001). Neurobiological research points to dysregulation in the amygdala, hippocampus, and prefrontal cortex, all of which are involved in emotion regulation and threat perception. Environmental factors such as trauma, childhood adversity, and chronic stress are also critical in the development of anxiety disorders. Cognitive models suggest that individuals prone to anxiety often engage in maladaptive thought patterns, such as catastrophizing, hypervigilance, and avoidance behaviors, which reinforce their anxious responses (Beck & Clark, 1997).

Anxiety is more than just a feeling; it is a whole-body response that involves intricate interactions between the brain, nervous system, and various physiological systems. Understanding the underlying mechanisms of anxiety provides a foundation for effective treatment and empowers individuals to take control of their mental health. With a combination of evidence-based therapies, self-awareness, and supportive environments, individuals can manage anxiety and lead fulfilling, balanced lives.

Understanding Depression and Anxiety

The Prevalence and Impact of Depression and Anxiety: A Statistical Overview Depression and anxiety are among the most common mental health disorders worldwide, affecting millions of individuals across different age groups, socioeconomic backgrounds, and cultures. These conditions not only impact personal well-being but also contribute to increased healthcare costs, reduced productivity, and a higher risk of developing other chronic illnesses. Understanding the prevalence and global impact of depression and anxiety is crucial for addressing these public health concerns effectively.

Global Prevalence of Depression and Anxiety

Depression and anxiety disorders affect a significant portion of the global population. According to the World Health Organization (WHO), more than 280 million people worldwide suffer from depression, making it one of the leading causes of disability (WHO, 2023). Anxiety disorders, which include generalized anxiety disorder (GAD), panic disorder, and social anxiety disorder, affect an estimated 301 million people globally, including 58 million children and adolescents (Institute for Health Metrics and Evaluation, 2021).

In the United States, depression and anxiety rates have been increasing over the past decade. The National Institute of Mental Health (NIMH) reports that approximately 21 million U.S. adults (8.3% of the population) experienced at least one major depressive episode in 2021 (NIMH, 2022). Among these, 64% experienced severe impairment in daily functioning, including work, relationships, and personal care. Anxiety disorders affect 40 million U.S. adults annually, representing 19.1% of the population, yet only 36.9% of individuals with anxiety disorders receive treatment (Anxiety and Depression Association of America, 2022).

Depression is more prevalent among women than men, with 10.3% of females experiencing major depressive episodes compared to 6.2% of males (NIMH, 2022). Anxiety disorders also disproportionately affect women, who are twice as likely to be diagnosed compared to men (Remes et al., 2016). The reasons for this disparity include hormonal differences, increased exposure to stressors, and variations in coping mechanisms.

Depression and Anxiety in Different Age Groups

Children and Adolescents

Mental health disorders often begin early in life. Studies indicate that one in five adolescents worldwide experiences a mental health disorder, with depression and anxiety being the most common (WHO, 2021). In the United States, 15.1% of adolescents aged 12–17 had a major depressive episode in 2021, with 27.0% of female adolescents affected compared to 11.8% of males (NIMH, 2022). Anxiety disorders in children and adolescents have also increased, with 31.9% of adolescents aged 13–18 meeting the criteria for an anxiety disorder diagnosis (Merikangas et al., 2010).

Young Adults and College Students

Young adults, particularly college students, are at high risk for depression and anxiety. According to a survey conducted by the American College Health Association (2022), 42% of college students reported symptoms of anxiety, while 36% experienced depression. Stress from academic pressure, social expectations, financial burdens, and uncertainty about the future contributes significantly to mental health struggles in this population.

Middle-Aged and Older Adults

Depression and anxiety in older adults are often underdiagnosed, yet they remain major public health concerns. Studies show that 7% of adults over 60 suffer from clinical depression, with social isolation, chronic illness, and loss of loved ones being key contributing factors (WHO, 2022). Anxiety disorders in older adults affect 10-20% of individuals, yet they are frequently mistaken for normal aging-related stress (Bryant et al., 2018).

The Economic and Social Burden of Depression and Anxiety
Depression and anxiety are not only leading causes of personal suffering but also have a profound economic and societal impact. The global economic burden of depression and anxiety disorders is estimated at $1 trillion annually due to lost productivity, absenteeism, and healthcare costs (Chisholm et al., 2016). In the United States, workplace absenteeism due to mental health conditions costs employers over $51 billion per year, with employees experiencing depression missing an average of 27 workdays annually (Stewart et al., 2003).

The link between mental health and chronic disease further exacerbates healthcare costs. Individuals with depression are more likely to suffer from cardiovascular disease, diabetes, and chronic pain conditions, leading to increased medical expenses and hospitalizations (Halaris, 2017). The risk of suicide is also significantly higher among those with untreated depression and anxiety, with depression being a factor in over 50% of suicides worldwide (WHO, 2023).

Mental Health Treatment and Barriers to Care

Despite the high prevalence of depression and anxiety, access to treatment remains a significant challenge. Studies show that over 75% of individuals with depression in low- and middle-income countries do not receive adequate treatment (WHO, 2023). Even in developed countries, barriers such as cost, stigma, lack of mental health professionals, and limited access to evidence-based therapies prevent individuals from seeking help (Patel et al., 2018). In the United States, nearly 60% of adults with mental illness do not receive treatment, with the highest rates of unmet needs occurring in rural areas where access to psychiatric care is limited (NIMH, 2022). Stigma also remains a major barrier, as individuals fear being labeled "weak" or "unstable" for seeking help (Corrigan & Watson, 2002).

The Biological Mechanisms of Depression and Anxiety

Depression and anxiety are influenced by a combination of genetic, environmental, and neurobiological factors. Research has shown that neurotransmitter imbalances, structural brain changes, hormonal dysfunction, and inflammation all contribute to these conditions (Feldman & Eidelman, 2020).

One of the most well-documented biological mechanisms involves neurotransmitter imbalances. Serotonin, dopamine, and norepinephrine are three key neurotransmitters involved in mood regulation. Serotonin (5-HT) is often referred to as the "happiness chemical" because it plays a vital role in stabilizing mood, improving sleep, and regulating emotions. Low serotonin levels have been linked to both depression and anxiety (Krishnan & Nestler, 2018). Dopamine (DA) is associated with motivation and reward. When dopamine levels are low, individuals experience anhedonia, which is a lack of pleasure and interest in life (Wise, 2020). Norepinephrine (NE) helps regulate the body's stress response, and imbalances in this neurotransmitter contribute to fatigue, mental fog, and heightened stress sensitivity (Moret & Briley, 2019).

Another critical system involved in depression and anxiety is the hypothalamic-pituitary-adrenal (HPA) axis, which regulates the body's stress response. Chronic stress leads to an overactive HPA axis, resulting in excessive release of cortisol, the body's primary stress hormone. High cortisol levels damage key areas of the brain, including the hippocampus, which is responsible for memory and mood regulation, and the prefrontal cortex, which governs rational thinking and decision-making (Gold et al., 2015). Dysfunction in this system contributes to persistent anxiety, emotional instability, and depressive symptoms (Pariante, 2017).

Recent research highlights the role of the gut-brain axis in mental health. The gut microbiome plays a significant role in neurotransmitter production and inflammation regulation. An imbalance in gut bacteria can lead to increased intestinal permeability ("leaky gut"), allowing inflammatory molecules to enter the bloodstream and reach the brain, further contributing to depression and anxiety (Clapp et al., 2017). Studies suggest that dietary interventions, probiotics, and fiber-rich foods can help restore gut microbiota balance and improve mental well-being (Foster et al., 2021).

Depression and anxiety are not one-size-fits-all conditions. They exist on a spectrum, with various subtypes affecting individuals differently. Understanding these distinctions is crucial for tailoring effective treatment approaches.

Types of Depression

- Major Depressive Disorder (MDD): Characterized by persistent sadness, loss of interest, fatigue, and sleep disturbances lasting at least two weeks (American Psychiatric Association, 2020).
- Persistent Depressive Disorder (PDD): Also known as dysthymia, this is a chronic form of depression lasting for two years or more, with milder but longer-lasting symptoms (Klein et al., 2020).
- Atypical Depression: Marked by mood reactivity, increased appetite, and excessive sleepiness (Singh & Gotlib, 2019).

- Bipolar Depression: A phase of bipolar disorder that alternates between depressive episodes and manic episodes (Grande et al., 2016).

The Physiological Changes in Depression and Anxiety

Several physiological changes occur in the brain and body when a person experiences depression and anxiety.

Structural Brain Changes

Studies have shown that chronic stress and prolonged depressive episodes lead to changes in brain structure.

- **Hippocampus shrinkage**: Chronic stress and high cortisol levels lead to a smaller hippocampus, impairing memory and emotional regulation (Sapolsky, 2015).
- **Prefrontal cortex dysfunction**: Reduced activity in this area weakens rational decision-making, focus, and emotional control (Arnsten, 2018).
- **Amygdala hyperactivity**: The amygdala, responsible for processing fear and emotions, becomes overactive, increasing anxiety and emotional reactivity (Etkin et al., 2019).
- **Chronic Inflammation and Oxidative Stress:** Depression and anxiety are associated with high levels of inflammation and oxidative stress. Increased pro-inflammatory cytokines such as IL-6, TNF-α, and CRP have been observed in individuals with depression, indicating a connection between immune system dysfunction and mood disorders (Miller & Raison, 2016). Oxidative stress damages neurons, worsening depressive symptoms and impairing brain function (Maes et al., 2020). Anti-inflammatory diets and omega-3 fatty acids have been found to reduce depressive symptoms by lowering systemic inflammation (Berk et al., 2019).

A Personal Perspective

For years, I lived with depression and PTSD, feeling as though I was trapped in my own mind. The statistics I have shared are not just numbers. They represent real people who, like me, struggled in silence. At the time, I had no idea that millions of others were experiencing the same overwhelming thoughts, exhaustion, and emotional numbness. It was only through research and self-discovery that I realized depression and anxiety are not just emotional struggles but complex biological conditions influenced by neurotransmitter imbalances, inflammation, and stress response dysregulation.

I also learned that recovery is possible. By addressing nutrition, lifestyle changes, stress management, and holistic healing, I was able to take control of my mental health. The numbers may seem daunting, but they also serve as a reminder that no one is alone in this battle. Understanding the prevalence, impact, and challenges of mental health disorders is the first step toward finding lasting solutions. No matter what treatments I tried, the symptoms kept returning, making everyday life feel overwhelming. It wasn't until I studied the science behind these conditions that I realized the importance of addressing root causes rather than simply managing symptoms. Depression and anxiety are not just psychological struggles but complex systemic conditions influenced by neurochemical imbalances, hormonal dysregulation, chronic inflammation, and environmental triggers. In the following chapters, I will share the 14 natural strategies that helped me heal, along with scientific evidence and practical steps to help you break free from depression and anxiety.

1. Food and Depression

Inflammatory Foods That Worsen Depression and Anxiety

The connection between food and mood is far more powerful than most people realize. In recent years, growing research has shown that the foods we eat not only fuel our bodies but also shape our emotional and cognitive well-being. While conventional approaches to treating depression often emphasize therapy and medication, nutritional psychiatry, a rapidly emerging field, reveals that diet plays a pivotal role in the onset, severity, and recurrence of depressive symptoms.

A groundbreaking study known as the SMILES trial (Jacka et al., 2017), published in *BMC Medicine*, was among the first randomized controlled trials to show that dietary improvement significantly reduced symptoms of major depressive disorder. Participants who adopted a diet rich in whole foods, vegetables, legumes, healthy fats, and proteins experienced a marked improvement in mood compared to those receiving only social support. This and other studies confirm what many holistic practitioners have long observed: nutrient-dense, anti-inflammatory diets can be just as effective, if not more, than pharmaceutical interventions in some cases.

Unfortunately, the standard Western diet, high in processed foods, refined carbohydrates, added sugars, and artificial ingredients, has been linked to chronic inflammation, blood sugar instability, gut dysbiosis, and neurochemical imbalances, all of which are risk factors for depression (Lassale et al., 2019; Marx et al., 2021). Poor nutrition doesn't just impact the body; it alters brain function, neurotransmitter production, and hormone regulation, silently undermining mental health from the inside out.

In this chapter, we'll explore how specific foods contribute to or protect against depression, how inflammation and gut health are connected to mood disorders, and which dietary patterns support long-term emotional balance. You'll also find practical strategies and tips for transitioning to a healing, anti-inflammatory diet that nourishes both your body and your brain.

1. Processed Sugar and High-Glycemic Foods

Diets high in refined sugar, white bread, and sugary beverages have been associated with an increased risk of depression and anxiety (Knüppel et al., 2017). High-glycemic foods cause rapid spikes and crashes in blood sugar levels, leading to mood swings, irritability, and increased stress hormone production. A study involving over 23,000 individuals found that those who consumed a high-sugar diet had a significantly higher risk of developing depression over a five-year period (Akbaraly et al., 2018).

Excess sugar consumption also promotes chronic inflammation, increases oxidative stress, and impairs brain-derived neurotrophic factor (BDNF), a protein essential for brain function and neuroplasticity (Rao et al., 2019).

2. Trans Fats and Unhealthy Processed Oils

Trans fats, commonly found in fried foods, margarine, and processed baked goods, have been linked to increased systemic inflammation and neuroinflammation. Studies suggest that diets high in hydrogenated oils and processed vegetable oils (such as soybean, canola, and corn oil) are associated with a higher risk of depression and cognitive decline (Gómez-Pinilla, 2019). A large-scale Mediterranean diet study found that individuals who consumed high amounts of trans fats had a 48% increased risk of depression compared to those who followed an anti-inflammatory diet rich in healthy fats like omega-3s (Sánchez-Villegas et al., 2019).

3. Artificial Sweeteners and Additives

Artificial sweeteners like aspartame, saccharin, and sucralose are often marketed as healthier alternatives to sugar, but research suggests they may have negative effects on mental health. Studies show that aspartame consumption reduces serotonin levels in the brain, increasing the risk of anxiety and depression (Walton et al., 2018).

Additionally, artificial food additives, including monosodium glutamate (MSG), food colorings, and preservatives, have been found to disrupt gut microbiota, increase oxidative stress, and contribute to mood disorders (Rana et al., 2021).

4. Processed Meats

Highly processed meats, such as hot dogs, sausages, and deli meats, contain high levels of sodium, nitrates, and preservatives, which have been linked to increased inflammatory markers in the body. A study published in *Molecular Psychiatry* found that individuals who consumed large amounts of processed meats had a 42% increased risk of developing depression (Jacka et al., 2017). Unprocessed meats in moderation can be part of a healthy diet, excessive consumption of processed meats combined with a low intake of antioxidant-rich fruits and vegetables contributes to inflammatory stress on the body and brain. (O'Neil et al., 2014).

5. Dairy Products with Added Hormones and Casein Sensitivity

Dairy products, particularly those containing added hormones and antibiotics, have been linked to hormonal imbalances and inflammatory responses that may worsen anxiety and depressive symptoms (Verduci et al., 2019). Additionally, some individuals experience casein sensitivity, which triggers inflammation and affects dopamine metabolism, potentially leading to mood disturbances (Lachance & Ramsey, 2015).

How Diet Affects the Gut-Brain Axis

Emerging research highlights the gut-brain connection, showing how the gut microbiome influences mental health. Unhealthy diets high in inflammatory foods reduce the diversity of beneficial gut bacteria, increasing the risk of gut permeability (leaky gut), which allows inflammatory toxins to enter the bloodstream and reach the brain (Cryan et al., 2019).

A 2017 clinical trial found that individuals who followed an anti-inflammatory diet for 12 weeks experienced a 32% reduction in depressive symptoms, supporting the significant role of diet in mental health. (Jacka et al., 2017). The study also showed that higher consumption of fiber, polyphenols, and omega-3s correlated with better mood outcomes.

A Personal Perspective

1. Food and Depression

For years, I unknowingly fueled my depression and anxiety with a diet high in processed sugars, unhealthy fats, and artificial additives. Despite trying various treatments, my symptoms persisted until I began removing inflammatory foods and adopting an anti-inflammatory diet. The change was profound. My energy levels improved, my mood stabilized, and my anxiety became more manageable.

Through years of research and clinical practice, I developed the ASTR Diet, a comprehensive nutritional approach designed to reduce inflammation, balance hormones, and support gut and brain health. The ASTR Diet focuses on anti-inflammatory, sustainable, toxin-free, and restorative foods to help the body heal naturally. It emphasizes whole, nutrient-dense foods such as organic vegetables, proteins, healthy fats, and fiber-rich carbohydrates while eliminating inflammatory foods like processed sugars, refined grains, artificial additives, and inflammatory oils.

Because the ASTR Diet is a complete lifestyle approach, it is difficult to cover all aspects in this chapter. For a detailed breakdown of the ASTR Diet and how it supports mental health, check out my book **Eat to Heal**, where I provide a step-by-step guide to using food as medicine to reduce inflammation, balance brain chemistry, and restore overall well-being.

The research is clear: what we eat directly affects our mental health. Eliminating inflammatory foods and replacing them with nutrient-dense, whole foods can significantly reduce neuroinflammation, support gut health, and regulate neurotransmitters.

EAT TO
HEAL

The ASTR Diet: Unlock the Healing Power of Food to End Sickness and Thrive

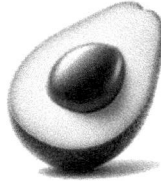

- Achieve Lasting Weight Loss
- Reverse Chronic Diseases Naturally
- Heal Inflammation and Pain
- Boost Energy and Vitality
- 3 Steps to Transform Your Health

Dr. Joseph Jacobs, DPT, ACN

2. Vitamins, Minerals & Hormones Imbalance

The Role of Vitamin and Mineral Deficiencies in Depression and Anxiety

For years, I struggled with depression, anxiety, chronic fatigue, and brain fog, searching for answers beyond temporary fixes. Through advanced lab testing, I discovered that I had eight key vitamin and mineral deficiencies, each playing a direct role in neurotransmitter function, hormone balance, and overall mental health. As I corrected these deficiencies, my symptoms gradually improved. Through my experience treating patients with chronic diseases, I have found that most individuals suffering from depression and anxiety have at least four to eight nutrient deficiencies, further highlighting the critical role of nutrition in mental health.

The Nutrient Deficiency Link: Challenging the Neurotransmitter Imbalance Theory of Depression

For decades, the dominant theory in psychiatry has held that depression is primarily the result of a chemical imbalance, specifically low levels of neurotransmitters like serotonin and dopamine. However, a growing body of evidence suggests this theory is both outdated and misleading. A review by Lacasse and Leo (2005) published in *PLoS Medicine* noted that while antidepressants are marketed as correcting a "chemical imbalance," no direct evidence has ever confirmed that people with depression have lower serotonin levels than those without. This undermines the foundational premise of many commonly prescribed medications and calls for a deeper investigation into the true causes of depression.

A critical, often overlooked factor in neurotransmitter production is the body's dependence on adequate levels of vitamins and minerals. Unlike neurotransmitters, which the body synthesizes internally, essential micronutrients must be obtained through diet or supplementation. For example, folate and vitamin B12 are crucial for methylation, a process necessary for neurotransmitter metabolism. A study by Almeida et al. (2005) found that low serum levels of folate and B12 were significantly associated with increased rates of depression in older adults. Similarly, a 2013 study published in the *Journal of Affective Disorders* linked low levels of magnesium, a cofactor in over 300 enzymatic reactions including those involved in serotonin production, to depressive symptoms (Tarleton et al., 2013).

Administering medications that artificially boost neurotransmitter activity without addressing these nutritional deficiencies may lead to short-term symptom relief but long-term dysfunction. SSRIs and other antidepressants work by forcing the release or prolonging the presence of neurotransmitters in the synaptic cleft, but if the body lacks the raw materials to replenish these chemicals, stores become depleted. This can result in diminishing drug effectiveness, dependency, withdrawal symptoms, and, paradoxically, increased suicidal thoughts and depressive episodes over time (Whitaker, 2010). This cycle reflects a failure to resolve the root cause of neurotransmitter imbalance: insufficient nutritional support.

As the field of nutritional psychiatry gains momentum, more studies support the integration of diet and supplementation into mental health treatment plans. A randomized controlled trial by Rucklidge et al. (2012) demonstrated that micronutrient supplementation significantly reduced symptoms of depression, anxiety, and stress compared to placebo in adults with mood disorders. Such findings highlight the importance of a foundational approach to mental health, one that prioritizes nutritional adequacy as the cornerstone of neurotransmitter health and emotional well-being.

Vitamins, Minerals, and Their Role in Neurotransmitter and Hormone Production

The human body requires 13 essential vitamins and at least 16 essential minerals to produce neurotransmitters and hormones crucial for mood regulation and emotional well-being. Key neurotransmitters such as serotonin and dopamine, commonly known as "happiness neurotransmitters," depend heavily on adequate levels of these nutrients. Serotonin synthesis, for example, requires vitamin B6, folate (vitamin B9), vitamin B12, magnesium, zinc, and iron, underscoring the intricate relationship between nutritional status and mental health (Kennedy, 2016). Similarly, dopamine synthesis relies significantly on adequate supplies of vitamins B6, B9, and minerals such as iron and copper, demonstrating that neurotransmitter balance is directly influenced by nutrient availability (Rucklidge & Kaplan, 2013).

Importantly, the human body cannot independently synthesize vitamins and minerals; therefore, obtaining sufficient amounts through diet or supplementation is crucial for maintaining hormonal and neurotransmitter balance. Deficiencies in these essential nutrients are associated with impaired production of neurotransmitters, subsequently increasing the risk of mood disorders such as depression. A study by Sánchez-Villegas et al. (2015) confirmed that dietary patterns rich in vitamins and minerals significantly lowered the incidence of depression, reinforcing the critical importance of nutritional adequacy in mood stabilization. This finding directly challenges the simplistic neurotransmitter imbalance theory of depression, highlighting that such imbalances are often symptoms of underlying nutritional deficiencies rather than isolated causes of mental health disorders.

Evaluating vitamin and mineral levels accurately is therefore crucial for addressing the root cause of depression rather than merely masking symptoms with pharmacological treatments targeting neurotransmitter systems. Rucklidge et al. (2017) emphasize the importance of thorough nutritional assessments, showing in clinical trials that comprehensive micronutrient supplementation effectively improved mood, reduced anxiety, and corrected neurotransmitter imbalances without the side effects commonly associated with psychiatric medications. These findings underscore the necessity of addressing nutritional deficits through proper evaluation and targeted interventions as a foundational approach to treating depression.

One of the biggest misconceptions about depression and anxiety is that they are simply caused by neurotransmitter imbalances, such as low serotonin and dopamine levels. While this theory has led to the widespread use of antidepressant medications like SSRIs, it fails to address a more fundamental issue: the body cannot produce neurotransmitters without the necessary vitamins and minerals. The human body is unable to create serotonin, dopamine, or norepinephrine out of nothing. It relies on specific nutrients to synthesize these critical brain chemicals. **The body cannot generate neurotransmitters unless it has access to the building blocks needed for their production and conversion.** If an individual is deficient in these essential nutrients, their neurotransmitter levels will remain low, regardless of how many medications they take.

Furthermore, because each person's deficiencies are unique, it is crucial to work with a clinical nutritionist to evaluate and properly dose the nutrients needed for recovery. If you suffer from depression or anxiety, there is a high probability that you have at least four to eight key nutrient deficiencies. The treatment must be customized to your individual needs, as excessive or imbalanced supplementation can be ineffective or even harmful.

Scientific research confirms that vitamin and mineral imbalances contribute to mood disorders, affecting brain chemistry, inflammation levels, and hormonal stability (Swardfager et al., 2013). This chapter will explore the most common deficiencies linked to depression and anxiety, their physiological effects, and how optimizing nutrient levels can support mental health recovery.

The Connection Between Nutrient Deficiencies and Mental Health

Nutrients play a fundamental role in neurotransmitter production, brain function, and hormonal regulation. Deficiencies in essential vitamins and minerals can lead to neurotransmitter imbalances, increased oxidative stress, inflammation, and mitochondrial dysfunction, all of which contribute to depression and anxiety (Mikkelsen et al., 2016).

Many individuals struggling with mental health conditions have low levels of vitamins such as B12, B6, D, and folate, as well as minerals like magnesium, zinc, and iron. These deficiencies impair the body's ability to produce serotonin, dopamine, and norepinephrine, which are critical for emotional stability, motivation, and stress regulation (Kaplan et al., 2015).

Chronic stress further depletes essential nutrients, worsening the cycle of fatigue, anxiety, and depression. Modern diets, high in processed foods and refined carbohydrates, fail to provide adequate amounts of these nutrients, leading to widespread deficiencies (Rao et al., 2020).

Key Vitamin Deficiencies That Contribute to Depression and Anxiety

1. Vitamin B12 (Cobalamin) Deficiency

Vitamin B12 is crucial for red blood cell formation, energy production, and neurotransmitter synthesis. A deficiency in B12 can lead to brain fog, fatigue, irritability, and depression. Studies show that individuals with low B12 levels are twice as likely to experience depression compared to those with optimal levels (Penninx et al., 2016). B12 is essential for methylation, a process that supports DNA repair and neurotransmitter production (Miller et al., 2020). Vegetarians, vegans, and individuals with digestive disorders (such as IBS or SIBO) are at higher risk of B12 deficiency (O'Leary & Samman, 2010). Excessive intake may cause numbness, burning sensations, and itching, emphasizing the need for personalized dosing.

2. Vitamin B6 (Pyridoxine) Deficiency

Vitamin B6 is necessary for the production of serotonin, dopamine, and GABA, which regulate mood, stress response, and cognitive function. Research indicates that low B6 levels are associated with increased anxiety, irritability, and depression (Hvas et al., 2004). B6 is also involved in homocysteine metabolism, and elevated homocysteine levels have been linked to higher rates of depression, cognitive decline and heart attack (Selhub et al., 2013). Excessive intake of vitamin B6 may lead to nerve damage, numbness, and tingling in the hands and feet, highlighting the importance of personalized dosing.

3. Folate (Vitamin B9) Deficiency

Folate is required for DNA synthesis and neurotransmitter function. Deficiency in folate has been associated with higher rates of depression, cognitive dysfunction, and poor response to antidepressants (Bender et al., 2017). A study found that patients with depression often have lower folate levels, and supplementation significantly improved symptoms (Young, 2013). Folate plays a key role in methylation and detoxification, supporting overall brain function (Bottiglieri, 2005).

4. Vitamin B3 (Niacin) Deficiency

Vitamin B3, also known as niacin, plays a crucial role in energy metabolism, neurotransmitter synthesis, and antioxidant defense. It is necessary for the production of NAD+ (nicotinamide adenine dinucleotide), a coenzyme essential for mitochondrial function and cellular energy production (Gowda et al., 2019). Low levels of NAD+ have been linked to fatigue, cognitive decline, and depressive symptoms.

A deficiency in niacin has been associated with neuropsychiatric symptoms, including irritability, apathy, and mood disorders. Severe deficiency can lead to pellagra, a condition characterized by dermatitis, diarrhea, and dementia, with depression being a primary symptom (Paranagama et al., 2018). While pellagra is rare in developed countries, subclinical niacin deficiency is more common than previously thought, particularly in individuals with chronic stress, poor diet, or high alcohol consumption (Gowda et al., 2019).

Studies suggest that niacin supplementation may help improve depressive symptoms by supporting serotonin production and reducing neuroinflammation (Wilkinson et al., 2018). Additionally, niacinamide, a form of vitamin B3, has been studied for its potential role in treating anxiety and depression, as it has neuroprotective and anti-inflammatory effects (Wilkinson et al., 2018).

5. Vitamin D Deficiency

Vitamin D acts as a hormone that regulates brain function, immune response, and inflammation. Deficiency has been strongly linked to seasonal affective disorder (SAD), depression, and anxiety. Studies show that low vitamin D levels increase the risk of depression by 50% (Anglin et al., 2013). Vitamin D deficiency reduces serotonin and dopamine production, which are essential for mood stability (Wilkins et al., 2016). Individuals living in low sunlight regions or spending excessive time indoors are more susceptible to low vitamin D levels (Ju et al., 2020). Optimal dosing requires lab-guided monitoring, as excessive vitamin D may lead to hypercalcemia, kidney strain, and increased cardiovascular risk.

6. Vitamin C Deficiency

Vitamin C, also known as ascorbic acid, is a potent antioxidant crucial for maintaining brain health, neurotransmitter synthesis, and overall emotional stability. Deficiencies in vitamin C have been increasingly linked to depressive symptoms, highlighting the importance of this nutrient in mental health.

According to research by Wang et al. (2013), low plasma vitamin C concentrations are associated with increased severity of depressive symptoms. This study indicated that individuals with lower levels of vitamin C were more likely to experience feelings of sadness, fatigue, and cognitive impairment compared to individuals with sufficient vitamin C levels.

Vitamin C plays an essential role in the synthesis of neurotransmitters, including serotonin and dopamine, both of which are involved in mood regulation.

Deficiency in vitamin C disrupts this synthesis, potentially contributing to depressive symptoms. For instance, a study conducted by Pullar, Carr, and Vissers (2017) demonstrated that increased intake of vitamin C could elevate mood, decrease anxiety, and improve emotional well-being, underscoring its therapeutic potential in depression management. Furthermore, due to its antioxidant properties, vitamin C helps reduce oxidative stress and inflammation, two factors strongly associated with depression. Lopresti, Hood, and Drummond (2015) found a clear relationship between higher dietary antioxidant intake, including vitamin C, and a lower risk of depression, suggesting that antioxidant-rich diets may protect against depressive symptoms.

Considering the substantial evidence linking vitamin C deficiency to depressive symptoms, ensuring adequate intake through dietary measures or supplementation is critical. Increasing consumption of vitamin C-rich foods such as citrus fruits, berries, leafy greens, and certain vegetables may provide therapeutic benefits for individuals experiencing depressive symptoms or at risk of depression due to nutrient deficiencies. Overall, addressing vitamin C deficiency represents a straightforward, low-risk approach to potentially alleviate depressive symptoms and enhance overall mental well-being.

7. Iron Deficiency

Iron is essential for oxygen transport, dopamine production, and energy metabolism. A deficiency in iron leads to fatigue, brain fog, and mood disturbances, which can mimic or worsen symptoms of depression and anxiety (Beard et al., 2008). Low iron levels impair the function of monoamine oxidase enzymes, which regulate serotonin and dopamine levels in the brain. Research shows that iron-deficient individuals are more likely to experience depressive symptoms, with women being particularly at risk due to menstruation and pregnancy-related iron loss (McClung & Karl, 2009).

A study published in *Psychiatry Research* found that iron deficiency anemia is associated with a 2.5 times greater risk of developing major depressive disorder (MDD) (Zhao et al., 2018). Iron is also necessary for myelin formation, which protects neurons and supports efficient neurotransmission. Deficiencies in iron lead to impaired cognitive function, poor concentration, and increased susceptibility to stress, all of which contribute to the severity of depressive episodes (Lozoff et al., 2013).

While iron supplementation is beneficial for those with diagnosed deficiency, excessive iron intake can increase oxidative stress, which may worsen inflammation. It is not safe to take iron supplements without laboratory testing to confirm a deficiency. This is why individualized lab testing and proper dosing by a clinical nutritionist are essential for correcting iron-related mood disorders.

8. Magnesium Deficiency

Magnesium is often referred to as the "relaxation mineral" because of its essential role in nervous system regulation, neurotransmitter function, and stress response. Low magnesium levels have been linked to higher rates of anxiety, irritability, and depression (Boyle et al., 2017). Magnesium regulates the function of the hypothalamic-pituitary-adrenal (HPA) axis, which controls the body's stress response. A deficiency can lead to excessive cortisol production, increasing the risk of chronic stress, emotional instability, and depressive symptoms (Tarleton et al., 2017).

A randomized controlled trial found that magnesium supplementation significantly improved depression scores within six weeks, making it an effective, natural alternative for managing depressive symptoms (Tarleton & Littenberg, 2017). Magnesium also plays a role in GABA (gamma-aminobutyric acid) production, an inhibitory neurotransmitter that promotes relaxation and helps counterbalance excessive excitatory signals in the brain. Low levels of GABA have been linked to panic attacks, restlessness, and persistent low mood (Eby & Eby, 2010).

Another critical function of magnesium is reducing neuroinflammation and oxidative stress, which are commonly elevated in individuals with depression. Studies suggest that people with low magnesium levels are at a higher risk of treatment-resistant depression, meaning they may not respond well to conventional antidepressants (Serefko et al., 2016). Given its broad role in brain function, restoring optimal magnesium levels through diet or supplementation can significantly improve symptoms of depression, anxiety, and chronic stress. Excessive intake may cause gastrointestinal symptoms, confusion, cardiac arrest, and kidney dysfunction, emphasizing the need for personalized dosing.

9. Zinc Deficiency

Zinc is a key mineral involved in brain plasticity, neurotransmitter regulation, and immune function. It plays an essential role in synaptic transmission and is found in high concentrations in the hippocampus, a brain region critical for memory, emotion regulation, and stress response (Nowak et al., 2018). Research shows that low zinc levels are strongly associated with depression, and individuals with lower zinc levels often have higher levels of inflammatory markers, suggesting that zinc deficiency contributes to neuroinflammation (Swardfager et al., 2013). A meta-analysis published in *Biological Psychiatry* found that individuals with low serum zinc levels were at a significantly higher risk of depression, and zinc supplementation improved depressive symptoms (Nowak et al., 2018). Zinc also influences glutamate and GABA activity, affecting mood stability and stress resilience.

Furthermore, zinc is involved in modulating the brain-derived neurotrophic factor (BDNF), a protein essential for neurogenesis and emotional regulation. Low BDNF levels have been linked to chronic stress, major depressive disorder, and cognitive impairment (Szewczyk et al., 2010). Given that zinc deficiency is common in individuals with chronic stress, correcting this deficiency through diet and supplementation may significantly improve depression, brain function, and emotional stability. It is not safe to take zinc supplements without laboratory testing to confirm a deficiency. Individualized lab testing and proper dosing by a clinical nutritionist are essential for correcting zinc-related mood disorders. Supplementation should be carefully monitored, as excessive zinc can lead to copper depletion and hormonal imbalances.

10. Iodine Deficiency

Iodine is a crucial micronutrient required for the production of thyroid hormones, which play a significant role in brain function and mood regulation. A deficiency in iodine can lead to hypothyroidism, a condition strongly associated with depressive symptoms. Research has shown that iodine deficiency, particularly during pregnancy, can have long-term effects on mental health. Bath, Steer, Golding, and Emmett (2013) found that inadequate iodine intake in pregnant women was linked to a higher risk of emotional difficulties, including depressive symptoms, in their children. Since the thyroid gland relies on iodine to synthesize thyroxine (T4) and triiodothyronine (T3), a deficiency in iodine can disrupt hormonal balance, leading to cognitive impairments and mood disorders (Zimmermann, 2012). Studies suggest that individuals with hypothyroidism often exhibit depressive symptoms, and restoring iodine levels can help improve mood and mental function. It is not safe to take iodine supplements without laboratory testing to confirm a deficiency. Individualized lab testing and proper dosing by a clinical nutritionist are essential for correcting iodine-related mood disorders.

11. Selenium Deficiency

Selenium is an essential trace element with strong antioxidant properties, helping to reduce oxidative stress and inflammation, both of which are associated with depression. Selenium plays a role in brain function by influencing neurotransmitter activity and protecting neurons from oxidative damage. A study by Pasco et al. (2012) found that individuals with lower selenium levels had a higher likelihood of developing major depressive disorder.

This aligns with evidence suggesting that oxidative stress contributes to depression, and selenium's role in antioxidant enzyme activity, such as glutathione peroxidase, may help counteract these effects. Additionally, a randomized controlled trial by Benton, Haller, and Fordyce (2016) demonstrated that selenium supplementation significantly improved mood and reduced depressive symptoms in participants with initially low selenium status. These findings highlight the importance of selenium in maintaining mental well-being and suggest that correcting selenium deficiency may be an effective strategy for alleviating depressive symptoms.

12. Coenzyme Q10 Deficiency

Coenzyme Q10 (CoQ10) is a vital nutrient that functions primarily within mitochondria to facilitate energy production and reduce oxidative stress, both critical processes for maintaining healthy brain function and emotional well-being. Emerging research has linked deficiencies in CoQ10 to depressive symptoms, suggesting its importance as a factor in mental health. According to a study by Morris et al. (2013), individuals suffering from depression often demonstrate lower serum levels of CoQ10 compared to healthy individuals, indicating that reduced CoQ10 availability might contribute to the onset or severity of depressive episodes.

The connection between CoQ10 and depression may be explained by its essential role in mitochondrial function and oxidative stress management. Depression has consistently been associated with mitochondrial dysfunction, reduced cellular energy metabolism, and increased oxidative stress. A randomized controlled trial by Forester et al. (2012) found that CoQ10 supplementation significantly reduced depressive symptoms and fatigue in patients with bipolar depression, providing compelling evidence of its potential as a therapeutic option. Additionally, another clinical trial conducted by Mehrpooya et al. (2018) demonstrated that CoQ10 supplementation not only improved mood but also enhanced cognitive performance and reduced oxidative stress markers in patients with depression.

These studies collectively suggest that addressing CoQ10 deficiency through dietary intervention or targeted supplementation may represent an effective strategy for managing depressive symptoms, especially in cases associated with mitochondrial dysfunction and increased oxidative stress. Including CoQ10-rich foods like organ meats, fatty fish, whole grains, nuts, and legumes, or considering supplementation, may offer benefits in supporting emotional resilience and overall mental health.

13. Omega-3 Fatty Acid Deficiency

Omega-3 fatty acids are essential fats critical for brain function, neurotransmitter activity, and the maintenance of healthy cell membranes. Deficiencies in omega-3 fatty acids, particularly docosahexaenoic acid (DHA) and eicosapentaenoic acid (EPA), have been consistently associated with depression and impaired mental health. A comprehensive review by Grosso et al. (2014) found strong evidence linking low omega-3 levels to increased risk of depressive disorders. The authors concluded that supplementation with EPA and DHA significantly reduced symptoms of depression, emphasizing the critical role omega-3 fatty acids play in mental well-being.

The neuroprotective and anti-inflammatory properties of omega-3 fatty acids appear to be central mechanisms underlying their beneficial effects on mood. Omega-3 fatty acids modulate neurotransmission, enhance neurogenesis, and reduce neuroinflammation, all of which contribute to their antidepressant properties. A meta-analysis conducted by Mocking et al. (2016) demonstrated that EPA supplementation, in particular, provided notable improvements in depressive symptoms, suggesting that targeted omega-3 supplementation could be a valuable therapeutic option. Additionally, Lin et al. (2010) observed that patients with major depressive disorder had significantly lower omega-3 concentrations in their blood compared to healthy controls, further supporting the relationship between omega-3 deficiency and depression.

Given these findings, addressing omega-3 fatty acid deficiency through dietary intake or supplementation may significantly benefit individuals experiencing depressive symptoms. Incorporating omega-3-rich foods, such as fatty fish (salmon, sardines), flaxseeds, chia seeds, walnuts, and fish oil supplements, can help mitigate depressive symptoms and support overall mental health.

Proper Evaluation for Better Outcomes

The Importance of Proper Evaluation Before Taking Supplements

Many people assume that taking vitamin and mineral supplements is always beneficial, but without proper evaluation, supplementation can do more harm than good. Before I studied nutrition and understood the importance of lab testing and individualized dosing, I made the mistake of taking supplements based on general recommendations rather than my specific needs.

Unfortunately, this led to unexpected side effects, including fatigue, digestive issues, and worsened mood symptoms. What I didn't realize at the time was that excessive or unbalanced intake of certain nutrients can create new deficiencies, disrupt biochemical pathways, and even increase inflammation.

For example, taking too much iron without confirmed deficiency can cause oxidative stress and damage tissues, while excessive zinc can deplete copper, leading to further imbalances. Similarly, high doses of vitamin B6 taken without medical supervision can lead to nerve toxicity and neuropathy (Spinneker et al., 2007). Magnesium supplements can also cause digestive discomfort or interfere with certain medications if taken improperly (Schwalfenberg & Genuis, 2017). These risks highlight why blind supplementation is not a safe or effective approach to improving health.

From both my personal experience and my clinical work, I have found that most individuals struggling with depression and anxiety have at least four to eight key nutrient deficiencies. However, the specific deficiencies and required dosages vary from person to person. This is why it is essential to work with a clinical nutritionist who can properly evaluate nutrient levels through lab testing and customize supplementation accordingly. The goal is to restore balance, not create new imbalances.

Taking the right supplements in the correct dosages can be life-changing, but guessing or following generic recommendations without professional evaluation can lead to wasted money, ineffective treatment, and even negative health effects. If you are struggling with depression or anxiety, I strongly encourage you to get tested, identify your specific deficiencies, and follow a tailored nutrition plan rather than experimenting with random supplements. A well-structured, individualized approach is the safest and most effective way to support your mental health and overall well-being.

A Personal Perspective

When I first began investigating the role of nutrients in mental health, I was shocked to discover that I had eleven key vitamin and mineral deficiencies. Despite eating what I thought was a healthy diet, I was lacking essential nutrients needed for neurotransmitter production, energy metabolism, and hormone balance. As I corrected these deficiencies, I noticed profound improvements in my mood, mental clarity, and overall well-being.

Through my experience treating patients with chronic diseases, I have observed that most individuals with depression and anxiety have at least four to eight nutrient deficiencies. Addressing these deficiencies through diet and targeted supplementation has been a game-changer in helping my patients regain their mental health. However, supplementation must be approached with precision and professional guidance. Working with a clinical nutritionist practitioner is essential to properly evaluate deficiencies and determine the correct dosage for each individual.

3. Drug-Induced Depression

Drug-Induced Depression: How Medications Can Trigger or Worsen Mood Disorders

For years, I struggled with depression and anxiety, searching for answers beyond temporary symptom management. While investigating the root causes of my condition, I discovered that certain medications can directly contribute to depression by altering brain chemistry, depleting essential nutrients, and disrupting hormone balance. What many people don't realize is that drug-induced depression is a well-documented phenomenon, yet it is often overlooked in both medical practice and mental health treatment.

Numerous studies have confirmed that medications prescribed for hypertension, pain management, hormonal imbalances, infections, and even mental health disorders can lead to depressive symptoms (Schatzberg et al., 2021). In many cases, these drugs interfere with neurotransmitter production, deplete essential vitamins and minerals, or cause systemic inflammation, all of which are linked to depression. This chapter explores the major categories of drugs that can cause depression, the mechanisms behind their effects, and what to do if you suspect that your medication is contributing to your mental health struggles.

Understanding Drug-Induced Depression

Drug-induced depression occurs when a medication disrupts brain chemistry, hormone regulation, or nutrient absorption, leading to depressive symptoms. These symptoms can develop soon after starting a medication or gradually over time. The severity varies depending on dosage, duration of use, individual susceptibility, and underlying health conditions (Fava et al., 2018).

The key mechanisms through which medications can induce depression include:

1. **Neurotransmitter Disruption:** Some drugs lower serotonin, dopamine, or norepinephrine levels, which can lead to low mood, fatigue, and apathy.
2. **Nutrient Depletion:** Certain medications deplete essential vitamins and minerals, such as B vitamins, magnesium, and zinc, that are necessary for neurotransmitter production.
3. **Hormonal Imbalance:** Medications that affect thyroid function, sex hormones, or cortisol levels may disrupt mood regulation.

3. Drug-Induced Depression

4. **Increased Inflammation:** Some drugs contribute to neuroinflammation, a process strongly linked to depression.

5.**Mitochondrial Dysfunction:** Certain medications interfere with cellular energy production, which may result in fatigue and cognitive decline.

Recognizing these effects is critical, as drug-induced depression is often misdiagnosed as a primary depressive disorder, leading to unnecessary psychiatric treatments instead of addressing the root cause (Viktorin et al., 2017).

Medications That Can Cause or Worsen Depression

1. **Cardiovascular Drugs** (Used for High Blood Pressure, Heart Disease, and Cholesterol)

Many commonly prescribed blood pressure and heart medications have been associated with depression due to their effects on neurotransmitter regulation, circulation, and nutrient depletion.
- Beta-Blockers (e.g., Propranolol, Metoprolol, Atenolol): These drugs lower norepinephrine and dopamine levels, leading to fatigue, lethargy, and low mood (Ko et al., 2021).
- Calcium Channel Blockers (e.g., Verapamil, Amlodipine): Can disrupt intracellular calcium balance, which is essential for neurotransmitter release and brain function (Furukawa et al., 2018).
- Statins (e.g., Atorvastatin, Simvastatin): Used for cholesterol management, statins can lower coenzyme Q10 (CoQ10) levels, leading to fatigue and brain fog (Gámez-Belmonte et al., 2020).

2. **Hormonal Medications** (Used for Birth Control, Menopause, and Thyroid Disorders)

Hormonal imbalances are a major contributor to mood disorders, and medications that alter hormone levels can lead to significant changes in mood stability and emotional regulation.

- Oral Contraceptives (e.g., Combination Birth Control Pills, Progestin-Only Pills): Studies show that hormonal birth control is linked to a 34% increased risk of depression, particularly in adolescents (Skovlund et al., 2016).

- Testosterone Blockers (e.g., Finasteride, Dutasteride): Used for prostate conditions and hair loss, these drugs interfere with androgen levels and have been linked to post-finasteride syndrome, characterized by persistent depression and cognitive impairment (Melcangi et al., 2017).
- Thyroid Medications (e.g., Levothyroxine, Methimazole): Both hypothyroidism and hyperthyroidism treatments can lead to mood instability, anxiety, and depressive symptoms if dosages are not well-balanced (Samuels et al., 2018).

3. **Pain Medications** (Used for Chronic Pain, Inflammation, and Migraines)
Pain medications, especially opioids, affect the brain's reward system and neurotransmitter balance, making individuals more susceptible to depression.

- Opioids (e.g., Morphine, Oxycodone, Hydrocodone, Tramadol): Long-term opioid use is linked to depression due to downregulation of dopamine receptors (Scherrer et al., 2016).
- NSAIDs (e.g., Ibuprofen, Naproxen, Diclofenac): While anti-inflammatory drugs can reduce pain, some studies suggest that chronic NSAID use may contribute to depressive symptoms by altering gut microbiota and immune function (Kaufmann et al., 2019).

4. **Neurological and Psychiatric Medications** (Used for Anxiety, Insomnia, and Seizures)

Ironically, some medications used to treat mental health and neurological disorders can actually induce or worsen depression.

- Benzodiazepines (e.g., Alprazolam, Lorazepam, Clonazepam): Often prescribed for anxiety and insomnia, benzodiazepines can cause rebound depression due to neurotransmitter depletion and dependency (Lader, 2011).
- Antiepileptic Drugs (e.g., Gabapentin, Pregabalin, Valproate, Topiramate): Commonly used for seizures and nerve pain, these drugs can disrupt GABA and glutamate balance, increasing the risk of depression (Verrotti et al., 2014).

5. **Antibiotics and Antimicrobials** (Used for Infections and Gut Health Conditions)

- Antibiotics can alter gut microbiota, leading to dysbiosis and reduced neurotransmitter production.
- Fluoroquinolones (e.g., Ciprofloxacin, Levofloxacin): These antibiotics have been associated with anxiety, depression, and suicidal ideation due to their impact on GABA receptors (Sharma et al., 2018).
- Anti-fungal Medications (e.g., Ketoconazole, Fluconazole): Some anti-fungal drugs affect cortisol metabolism, leading to mood changes (Labad et al., 2018).

A Personal Perspective

Before I began studying clinical nutrition and functional medicine, I was unaware of the connection between medications and depression. Like many others, I assumed that my symptoms were purely biochemical or emotional, without considering how certain medications might be affecting my brain chemistry, gut health, and hormonal balance.

Through personal experience and working with patients suffering from chronic diseases and mental health conditions, I have found that many individuals unknowingly develop depression as a side effect of their medications. In these cases, the key to recovery is identifying and addressing the root cause rather than simply adding another medication to the mix.

If you suspect that a medication may be contributing to your depression, it is important to work with your healthcare provider to evaluate alternative options. Medication-induced depression is often reversible, and by optimizing nutrient levels, reducing inflammation, and addressing medication side effects, many individuals can regain their mental well-being.

4. Brain Glitches: Your Thoughts Are Not You

Your Thoughts Are Not You: Understanding Brain Glitches, Hallucinations, and Irrational Thoughts

For years, I struggled with intrusive thoughts, irrational fears, and overwhelming anxiety. These thoughts would appear suddenly, often making no logical sense, yet they felt real and emotionally intense. I used to believe that these thoughts defined me. But through years of research and clinical experience, I learned a profound truth: your thoughts are not you. The human brain, while an incredible organ, is prone to glitches, misfires, and distortions in perception. Just because a thought appears in your mind does not mean it is true or reflective of reality.

Understanding how irrational thoughts, brain glitches, and hallucinations occur can help you separate yourself from them, reducing their emotional impact. This chapter explores why these thoughts happen, how they are formed, and what you can do to break free from their influence.

Why Do We Experience Irrational Thoughts?

The human brain processes millions of pieces of information every second, filtering what is relevant and discarding what is not. However, sometimes errors in processing, misinterpretations, or past traumas can cause irrational thoughts to surface. These thoughts may appear in the form of self-doubt, paranoia, obsessive fears, or even hallucinations (Brewin et al., 2010).

Several key factors contribute to the emergence of irrational thoughts:

1. **The Brain's Pattern Recognition System**: The brain is wired to detect patterns and threats, even when none exist. This mechanism evolved as a survival strategy but can lead to false alarms, such as assuming someone dislikes you based on a neutral expression (Gilbert, 1998).
2. **Hyperactive Amygdala** (Fear Center of the Brain): The amygdala is responsible for detecting threats and triggering the fight-or-flight response. When overactive, it can create irrational fears and anxiety-driven thoughts (LeDoux, 2015).
3. **Cognitive Distortions:** These are thinking errors that make irrational thoughts seem real, such as catastrophizing, black-and-white thinking, or mind-reading (Burns, 1989).

4. **Neurotransmitter Imbalances:** Low levels of serotonin and dopamine can affect emotional regulation, leading to repetitive negative thoughts, intrusive worries, and even hallucinations (Millan et al., 2012).

These glitches occur because the brain is not always operating in a perfectly logical manner. Instead, it relies on previous experiences, emotional states, and survival mechanisms, which can sometimes lead to false or irrational conclusions.

Rumination: The Mental Loop That Fuels Emotional Distress

Rumination is a psychological process in which a person repeatedly and passively focuses on the same distressing thoughts, problems, or feelings without moving toward resolution. It is not the same as healthy reflection or problem solving. Instead, rumination traps the mind in a loop of negativity, often amplifying emotional pain and reinforcing helplessness.

In depression, rumination typically centers on themes of worthlessness, past failures, or hopelessness about the future. A person might find themselves constantly replaying painful memories or asking, *"Why am I like this?"* without gaining any new insight. This cycle of repetitive, self-critical thinking deepens depressive symptoms and prevents emotional healing.

In anxiety disorders, rumination often takes the form of excessive worry about potential future threats or the consequences of past actions. The mind continually rehearses worst-case scenarios, leading to chronic stress and hypervigilance. Unlike productive planning, this type of mental activity is circular and emotionally draining, increasing physiological symptoms like restlessness, muscle tension, and insomnia.

In post-traumatic stress disorder (PTSD), rumination is frequently linked to unresolved trauma. Individuals may mentally relive the traumatic event, replaying images, emotions, and perceived mistakes. The brain fails to process the experience as something that occurred in the past and instead treats it as if it is still happening. This chronic reactivation of fear pathways keeps the nervous system stuck in survival mode and blocks recovery.

Neuroscientifically, rumination is associated with heightened activity in the default mode network (DMN), a brain system involved in self-referential thought and internal focus. At the same time, the prefrontal cortex, responsible for emotional regulation and perspective taking, becomes less effective, especially in those with mood and anxiety disorders. This neurological imbalance can be described as a brain glitch, a pattern of misfiring or overactivation that perpetuates suffering even when no real threat or problem exists in the moment.

These repetitive thought loops are not a character flaw; they are a malfunction in how the brain processes stress and emotion. Recognizing rumination as a brain-based phenomenon, rather than a reflection of truth, empowers individuals to respond with compassion, awareness, and effective tools for change.

Brain Glitches: When Your Mind Plays Tricks on You

The brain is an advanced predictive machine, constantly guessing what will happen next based on past experiences and limited sensory input. However, this predictive ability is not perfect, leading to cognitive errors, memory distortions, and even hallucinations.

1. False Memories and Misinterpretations

Have you ever been absolutely sure about a past event, only to find out later that your memory was incorrect? This is because memory is not a perfect recording but a reconstruction that is influenced by emotions, suggestions, and expectations (Loftus & Palmer, 1974). False memories can create unnecessary guilt, fear, or anxiety about things that never actually happened.

2. The Inner Critic and Negative Thought Loops

The prefrontal cortex, responsible for rational thinking, sometimes creates self-critical narratives based on past failures or perceived weaknesses. These thought loops are often exaggerated, making people believe they are not good enough, incapable, or destined to fail, even when there is no objective evidence to support these beliefs (Beck, 1976).

3. Perceptual Distortions and Mild Hallucinations

Hallucinations are often associated with psychiatric disorders, but mild hallucinations and perceptual distortions are much more common than people realize. Stress, sleep deprivation, sensory overload, and even anxiety can trick the brain into misperceiving reality (Waters et al., 2014).
Examples include:

- Hearing your name being called when no one is around
- Seeing shadows or movements in your peripheral vision
- Feeling like you are being watched when alone

These experiences are not signs of insanity but rather the brain misinterpreting incomplete sensory information.

Why Irrational Thoughts Feel Real

The reason irrational thoughts feel real is because they activate the same neurological and emotional pathways as real experiences. For example, if you suddenly think, *"What if I lose control and say something inappropriate?"*, your brain may react as if this is actually happening, triggering feelings of anxiety and distress.

This happens because of three main factors:

1. The Brain's Emotional Response: The brain treats imagined scenarios as if they are actual experiences, releasing stress hormones like cortisol and adrenaline (Brosschot et al., 2006).
2. Cognitive Fusion: This is when people fuse their identity with their thoughts, believing that *"If I think it, it must be true"* (Hayes et al., 1999).
3. Overactive Default Mode Network (DMN): The DMN, responsible for self-referential thinking, is hyperactive in individuals with anxiety and depression, causing overanalysis and excessive self-focus (Sheline et al., 2009).

How to Break Free from Irrational Thoughts

Recognizing that your thoughts are not you is the first step toward gaining control over them. Here are key strategies to detach from irrational thoughts and rewire your brain:

1. Identify Cognitive Distortions: When an irrational thought arises, ask yourself:
   - *Is this thought based on fact or fear?*
   - *What evidence supports or contradicts this thought?*
   - *How would I view this situation if I were calmer or advising a friend?*
2. Practice Mindfulness and Thought Defusion: Mindfulness helps you observe thoughts without attaching to them. Instead of saying *"I am a failure,"* reframe it as *"I am having a thought that I am a failure."* This small shift reduces emotional impact (Kabat-Zinn, 1994).
3. Regulate Your Nervous System: Deep breathing, progressive muscle relaxation, and vagus nerve stimulation calm the amygdala and reduce the emotional charge of irrational thoughts (Porges, 2011).
4. Address Neurotransmitter Balance: Since low levels of serotonin, dopamine, and GABA can contribute to intrusive thoughts and anxiety, addressing vitamin and mineral deficiencies, gut health, and inflammation can help restore emotional balance (Young, 2007).
5. Challenge Hallucinations and Perceptual Distortions: If you experience mild auditory or visual distortions, remind yourself that the brain is wired to fill in gaps of perception. Most perceptual errors occur under stress or fatigue, and grounding techniques can help differentiate reality from illusion.

Understanding the Nature of Thoughts

The human brain is an intricate network of electrical and chemical processes that generate thoughts continuously. However, what many fail to recognize is that thoughts are not always grounded in reality. Neuroscientific studies suggest that thoughts are often hallucinatory loops of the brain, meaning they are internally generated perceptions rather than direct reflections of the external world (Corlett, Honey, & Fletcher, 2007). This phenomenon explains why individuals can experience intrusive, irrational, or even distressing thoughts that have no factual basis. Recognizing this nature of thought allows people to disengage from automatic mental patterns and avoid over-identifying with their internal dialogue.

The Brain's Hallucinatory Nature of Thought Processing

Research in predictive coding theory suggests that the brain constantly generates predictions about reality based on past experiences rather than simply reacting to new information (Friston, 2010). This means that much of what people perceive, including their thoughts, is a projection of internally generated patterns rather than an objective representation of the present moment. A study by Powers et al. (2017) found that individuals prone to strong cognitive biases, such as anxiety or paranoia, are more likely to experience thought loops that function similarly to hallucinations. This occurs because the brain's default mode network (DMN), which governs self-referential thinking and mind-wandering, is hyperactive in people who struggle with negative thinking patterns (Buckner, Andrews-Hanna, & Schacter, 2008). Essentially, the DMN creates a self-generated feedback loop where a single negative thought reinforces itself, much like an echo chamber in the mind.

Moreover, research using fMRI brain imaging shows that when individuals are lost in thought, their brain activity is strikingly similar to that of individuals experiencing mild hallucinations (Alderson-Day & Fernyhough, 2015). This suggests that many of the thoughts people assume to be "true" are simply internally generated illusions that may have no correlation with external reality.

Cognitive Distortions and Thought Loops

Many psychological disorders, including obsessive-compulsive disorder (OCD), anxiety, and depression, are characterized by maladaptive thought loops that function as self-sustaining hallucinations. For example, in OCD, individuals experience recurrent intrusive thoughts, such as fears of contamination or doubts about safety, which trigger compulsive behaviors (Szechtman & Woody, 2004). The brain misinterprets these intrusive thoughts as genuine threats, despite no actual danger. This reinforces a hallucinatory loop of fear and compulsion that distorts reality.

Similarly, individuals suffering from rumination, a hallmark of depression, experience repetitive negative thoughts that mimic self-induced hallucinations (Nolen-Hoeksema, Wisco, & Lyubomirsky, 2008). The more a person engages with these thoughts, the more real they feel, despite their lack of factual grounding. This phenomenon explains why some individuals feel trapped in cycles of self-doubt, worry, or despair even when their external circumstances do not warrant such distress.

The **Reticular Activating System (RAS)** is a complex network of neurons located in the brainstem that plays a crucial role in filtering sensory information and regulating consciousness, attention, and alertness. The human brain is constantly processing vast amounts of sensory input, but it is impossible to consciously register all of this information at once. The RAS serves as a gatekeeper, determining what stimuli reach our conscious awareness based on relevance to our goals, beliefs, and emotions (Moruzzi & Magoun, 1949). For example, if a person is in a noisy environment but someone mentions their name, the RAS prioritizes that information, bringing it to their attention. This selective focus mechanism allows individuals to navigate their surroundings efficiently without being overwhelmed by unnecessary details.

The **RAS is programmed by repeated focus and belief patterns**, meaning that what a person consistently thinks about influences what their brain perceives as important. This is known as selective attention, a phenomenon supported by cognitive psychology research (Raz & Buhle, 2006). If an individual frequently thinks about success, personal growth, and opportunities, their RAS will filter in more experiences and evidence that align with these thoughts. For example, someone actively seeking a job may suddenly notice job openings and networking opportunities that they previously overlooked. This effect is also seen in marketing; when a person considers purchasing a particular car model, they start noticing that car everywhere because their RAS has heightened sensitivity to that specific stimulus.

Conversely, when an individual **focuses on fear, failure, or scarcity**, their RAS reinforces these perceptions by filtering in experiences that validate their negative expectations. Neuroscientific research indicates that chronic stress and negative thinking can create cognitive biases that shape how individuals perceive their reality (Baumeister et al., 2001). For instance, if a person believes they will fail an exam, their RAS may heighten awareness of past mistakes or difficulties, reinforcing feelings of inadequacy. This self-reinforcing cycle can make it difficult to break free from negative thinking patterns, which is why intentional mental and physical shifts are essential.

Reprogramming the **RAS through mindset and behavior changes** can help individuals notice opportunities, solutions, and synchronicities that align with their goals. Studies in neuroplasticity suggest that the brain's neural pathways can be rewired through repeated thought patterns and behaviors (Doidge, 2007).

The Role of Mindfulness and Cognitive Defusion

One of the most effective ways to break free from thought-induced hallucinations is through cognitive defusion, a technique used in Acceptance and Commitment Therapy (ACT) (Hayes, Strosahl, & Wilson, 1999). Cognitive defusion teaches individuals to observe thoughts as mental events rather than truths, allowing them to disengage from self-generated distortions.

Additionally, mindfulness meditation has been shown to deactivate the DMN and reduce the tendency for the brain to create thought loops (Brewer et al., 2011). Studies indicate that experienced meditators have significantly lower DMN activity, making them less prone to over-identifying with thoughts (Garrison et al., 2015). By practicing mindfulness, individuals learn to witness thoughts without attaching meaning to them, breaking the cycle of mental illusions.

Practical Strategies to Detach from Thought Loops

To reduce the impact of thought-generated hallucinations, individuals can implement the following strategies:

1. Cognitive Defusion: Label thoughts as "just thoughts" rather than believing them as truths (Hayes et al., 1999).
2. Mindfulness Practices: Engage in meditation to train the brain to disengage from thought loops (Brewer et al., 2011).
3. Reality Checking: Question the validity of thoughts instead of assuming they reflect reality (Freeman et al., 2017).
4. Breath Awareness: Using deep breathing exercises can shift focus away from the mind's hallucinations and into the present moment (Zeidan et al., 2010).

One of the most empowering realizations in overcoming depression is this: your thoughts are not always true. During depressive episodes, the brain often generates what can be called "brain glitches," automatic, distorted thoughts that reinforce negativity, hopelessness, and fear. These thoughts may feel convincing, but they are often exaggerated or completely false. Recognizing and discrediting them is the first step toward healing.

Fueling the Fire vs. Extinguishing It

Imagine your mind like a fireplace. When you dwell on these brain glitches by entertaining them, analyzing them, or emotionally reacting, you're pouring gasoline on the fire, which intensifies your emotional distress. However, when you pause, observe the thought from a distance, and simply say, "This is just a glitch, not reality," you are pouring water on the fire. Mindfulness-based cognitive therapy supports this approach by teaching individuals to observe thoughts without judgment, which has been shown to reduce rumination and depressive symptoms (Segal, Williams, & Teasdale, 2013).

Distorted Glasses: Challenging Cognitive Distortions

Another helpful metaphor is to imagine brain glitches as distorted glasses. If you wear glasses with warped lenses, your entire world will appear skewed. Similarly, when you interpret life through the lens of negative automatic thoughts, everything feels more threatening, hopeless, or pointless than it truly is. But once you discredit those thoughts, it's like removing the distorted glasses, allowing you to see reality more clearly.

Horse's Bit: Regaining Control

A third image to consider is the horse's bit, a small tool that can direct the path of a powerful animal. Your thoughts function similarly. If you allow hallucinated, glitchy thoughts to guide you, you may unknowingly follow an illusion, veering far from reality. You might be led by shame, fear, or despair that doesn't match your actual circumstances. But when you step back, examine the thought, and challenge it, you take the reins back and redirect your life toward truth and healing. Research supports that changing one's relationship with thoughts leads to better emotional regulation and long-term recovery (Kazantzis et al., 2018).

In short, your thoughts have power only when you believe them. Learn to question them; not every thought deserves your trust.

A Personal Perspective

Before I understood how the brain misinterprets information and generates false narratives, I felt trapped by my thoughts. I believed that every negative thought I had meant something about me, and I struggled with self-doubt, guilt, and anxiety because of it. Learning that the brain is imperfect and prone to glitches helped me realize that my thoughts were not always a reflection of reality.

Through my research and clinical experience, I have seen countless patients suffering from irrational thoughts, obsessive fears, and mild hallucinations, convinced that something was wrong with them. The truth is, these experiences are often the result of biochemical imbalances, cognitive distortions, and environmental stressors, not a reflection of their character or reality.

By understanding how the brain processes information and why irrational thoughts arise, you can begin to detach from them, reframe them, and take back control of your mental well-being.

Conclusion

The idea that "Your Thoughts Are Not You" is supported by neuroscience, psychology, and cognitive research. Thoughts are often hallucinatory loops of the brain, generated by predictive mechanisms rather than factual evidence. Over-identification with thoughts leads to cognitive distortions, stress, and mental health challenges. However, by understanding that thoughts are merely mental constructs, individuals can develop greater emotional resilience and clarity. Through cognitive defusion, mindfulness, and reality-checking strategies, people can break free from thought-induced illusions and live with greater mental freedom.

5. Distance Yourself & Zoom Out

Why Fighting Negative Thoughts Makes Them Stronger, and How Cognitive Defusion Can Set You Free

When we experience painful or self-critical thoughts, such as "I'm not good enough," "I always fail," or "Nothing will ever get better," our natural reaction is often to push back. We try to reason with ourselves, replacing the negative thought with something more rational or positive. On the surface, this seems like a logical strategy. However, research increasingly shows that this effort to "talk yourself out of" a negative thought can actually make things worse.

The problem lies in how the brain interprets attention and engagement. Neuroscience has shown that the more we focus on or repeat a thought, whether we are agreeing with it or trying to refute it, the more we reinforce the underlying neural pathway. According to Kross and Ayduk (2011), repeatedly engaging with distressing thoughts, even in an attempt to challenge them, can deepen rumination and increase emotional reactivity. This occurs because the brain assumes that what you engage with is important. Therefore, by arguing with negative thoughts, we unintentionally validate them as truths worth addressing. Over time, this strengthens their neural connections, making these thoughts more automatic and persistent.

This is further supported by the concept of neuroplasticity, the brain's ability to change its wiring based on experience and repetition. **Every time you argue with a negative thought, you reinforce its structure in the brain**, essentially telling your nervous system, *"This matters. Keep it active."* This can create a more permanent and reactive network that makes future negative thoughts more likely to arise and harder to dismiss. Instead of weakening the thought, this internal dialogue often results in entrenching it more deeply.

In contrast, a more effective approach comes from cognitive defusion, a core process in Acceptance and Commitment Therapy (ACT). Cognitive defusion involves stepping back and observing your thoughts as temporary mental events rather than truths. One powerful defusion strategy is to label these recurring negative thoughts as **brain glitches**, brief misfires in neural processing, not reflections of your identity or reality. When we see thoughts this way, we strip them of their emotional weight and avoid reinforcing them through internal conflict.

Instead of thinking, *"I'm worthless,"* and trying to replace it with *"No, I'm valuable,"* you might instead say, *"That's just a brain glitch."* This small reframing act distances you from the thought and helps prevent it from embedding deeper into memory. Studies on emotional labeling and distancing have shown that this approach reduces activity in the amygdala (the brain's emotional center) and increases activation in the prefrontal cortex, which supports rational thinking and self-regulation (Lieberman et al., 2007; Ochsner et al., 2002).

Labeling thoughts as glitches may seem subtle, but it's neurologically powerful. It shifts your relationship with your inner dialogue from resistance to observation. Over time, this decreases the brain's tendency to cling to negative thought patterns and allows for synaptic pruning, a process where unused neural pathways weaken and fade. Rather than reinforcing the thought, you allow it to pass without resistance or judgment.

In summary, while it may feel helpful to counter negative thoughts with logic or affirmations, doing so can reinforce their presence and build lasting networks in the brain. A more effective and scientifically grounded alternative is cognitive defusion. By acknowledging these thoughts as nothing more than brain glitches, temporary mechanical misfires, you can weaken their grip and free your mind from the cycle of internal conflict. This shift empowers you to reduce the emotional weight of negative thinking and reclaim control over your mental well-being.

What Is Cognitive Defusion?

Cognitive defusion is a psychological technique used in Acceptance and Commitment Therapy (ACT) to help individuals detach from their thoughts rather than being controlled by them (Hayes, Strosahl, & Wilson, 1999). It is based on the idea that thoughts are just words, images, or mental events, not absolute truths or direct reflections of reality. The goal of cognitive defusion is to reduce the power of negative or unhelpful thoughts by changing how individuals interact with them, rather than trying to eliminate or suppress them.

How Cognitive Defusion Works

Cognitive defusion techniques encourage individuals to:

1. **Observe thoughts without judgment:** Instead of reacting emotionally, individuals can learn to step back and view thoughts as passing mental events.
2. **Label thoughts for what they are:** For example, instead of thinking, "I'm a failure," one can reframe it as, "I'm having the thought that I'm a failure." This simple shift creates psychological distance and helps prevent over-identification with the thought
3. **Use humor or exaggeration:** Repeating a negative thought in a funny voice or turning it into a silly phrase can help reduce its emotional intensity.
4. **Visualize thoughts as separate from oneself:** Some exercises encourage individuals to imagine their thoughts floating by like leaves on a stream or clouds in the sky, reinforcing the idea that thoughts are temporary and not necessarily important.

Scientific Evidence Supporting Cognitive Defusion

Research shows that cognitive defusion reduces psychological distress and improves emotional regulation. A study by Masuda et al. (2004) found that individuals who practiced cognitive defusion experienced less distress from negative self-referential thoughts compared to those who engaged in thought suppression. Another study by Heppner et al. (2018) demonstrated that cognitive defusion techniques lower emotional reactivity and increase psychological flexibility, making individuals more resilient to stress.

Brain imaging studies suggest that cognitive defusion helps deactivate overactivity in the default mode network (DMN), a brain region associated with repetitive self-referential thinking (Brewer et al., 2011). This supports the idea that defusing from thoughts reduces mental chatter and promotes present-moment awareness.

Cognitive Defusion vs. Cognitive Restructuring

Unlike cognitive restructuring (used in Cognitive Behavioral Therapy), which focuses on changing negative thoughts into more rational ones, cognitive defusion emphasizes changing the relationship with thoughts rather than their content. This means that individuals do not have to fight or argue with negative thoughts; instead, they learn to observe them without being emotionally affected.

Real-Life Example of Cognitive Defusion

Imagine someone preparing for a presentation who has the thought, "I'm going to embarrass myself." Instead of believing this thought and feeling anxious, they apply cognitive defusion:

- They acknowledge, "I'm noticing the thought that I'm going to embarrass myself."
- They imagine the thought as a sentence written on a cloud, floating away.
- They say the thought in a cartoon voice to make it seem less threatening.

By doing this, they disempower the thought and prevent it from controlling their emotions and behavior.

Cognitive defusion is a powerful tool for improving mental resilience, emotional regulation, and stress management. By learning to step back and observe thoughts rather than identifying with them, individuals can reduce anxiety, depression, and overthinking. Research continues to support its effectiveness, making it an essential component of psychological well-being.

Distancing Yourself from Irrational Thoughts: How to Zoom Out and Regain Control

For years, I felt trapped by my thoughts. Every irrational worry, every intrusive fear, every doubtful scenario felt so real that I would react emotionally as if these thoughts were absolute truth. It wasn't until I learned to distance myself from irrational thoughts that I realized something profound: just because a thought appears in your mind does not mean it is real, meaningful, or worth your energy.

The key to managing irrational thoughts is not to argue with them, fight them, or suppress them; this only fuels them. Instead, the goal is to observe them without engaging, to zoom out, detach, and let them pass without allowing them to dictate your emotions or actions.

Your Thoughts Are Like a Movie: Watch, Don't Act

One of the simplest ways to distance yourself from irrational thoughts is to treat them like a movie playing on a screen. Imagine sitting in a theater, watching a dramatic, over-the-top film filled with exaggerated fears and negative predictions. You are not inside the movie, you are just watching it unfold. You can acknowledge that the storyline is intense and emotional, but at the same time, you understand that it's just a movie, not reality.

This same approach applies to irrational thoughts. When an anxious or irrational thought appears, instead of jumping into the storyline and acting as if it's real, remind yourself:

- *"This is just a thought, not a fact."*
- *"I am watching my brain create a dramatic scene, but I don't have to participate."*
- *"Just like a movie, this thought will pass and end on its own."*

By shifting your perspective to that of an observer, you create mental space between you and your thoughts, reducing their emotional impact.

Ask Yourself: Is This Thought Worth My Energy?

When an irrational thought pops up, I sometimes take a step back and literally talk to myself:
- *"Are you serious? This is a crazy thought!"*
- *"Here's another example of a brain glitch"*
- *"If I heard someone else say this, would I believe them?"*
- *"Would this thought matter in a week or a year?"*

This simple questioning immediately reduces the power of the thought. It allows you to recognize when a thought is irrational, exaggerated, or completely unfounded, making it easier to dismiss.

Campfire

Imagine your mind as a campfire, and every time you entertain an irrational thought, you add more fuel to the fire, making it grow stronger. The goal is to do the opposite: to pour water on the fire by depriving it of energy. The more you detach, question, and minimize the importance of irrational thoughts, the weaker they become.

The Zoom-Out Method: Expanding Your Perspective

Irrational thoughts often feel overwhelming because they take up all the space in your mind, making it hard to see the bigger picture. A useful technique to break free from this tunnel vision is zooming out, mentally stepping back to see your thoughts in a wider context. Here are several practical techniques for zooming out, or using cognitive defusion, from irrational thoughts.

1. The Google Earth Perspective

Imagine looking at your life through Google Earth. Right now, your irrational thought feels huge because you are zoomed in at street level, focusing only on this moment. But what happens when you zoom out?

• Look at your entire week: is this thought still as significant?
• Look at your whole year: will this thought still matter?
• Look at your whole life: is this just a passing blip in a much bigger picture?

When you shift your focus beyond the present moment, irrational thoughts shrink in importance, making them easier to let go.

2. The Friend Perspective

If a friend came to you with the same irrational thought you are having, how would you respond? Would you agree with their fear, or would you help them see a more rational perspective?

By imagining your thought coming from someone else, you naturally distance yourself from it, making it easier to assess rationally instead of emotionally.

3. The Third-Person Perspective

Instead of thinking *"I am anxious"*, reframe it as *"My brain is experiencing anxiety right now"*. This small shift creates distance between you and your emotions, helping you recognize that feelings are temporary and separate from your identity.

4. Let Thoughts Drift Away Like Clouds

Another powerful way to detach from irrational thoughts is to visualize them as clouds floating across the sky.
- When a thought appears, acknowledge it without resistance; don't push it away, but don't hold onto it either.
- Imagine placing the thought on a passing cloud and watching it drift away.
- Remind yourself that thoughts are temporary, just like clouds; they appear, move across your mind, and then disappear.

This technique helps reinforce that thoughts are not permanent, not defining, and not always meaningful.

5. Labeling the Thought: "Oh, It's Just That Again"

One mistake I used to make was treating every irrational thought as if it were a brand-new crisis that needed my attention. But in reality, most irrational thoughts are recycled fears, worries, or insecurities that my brain keeps reusing. Instead of engaging with these thoughts, I started labeling them:

- *"Oh, it's just my anxiety talking again."*
- *"Here's that silly thought I always get when I'm tired."*
- *"This is just my brain being dramatic."*

Labeling helps reduce the urgency of irrational thoughts, making them feel less powerful and easier to ignore.

6. Shift from Thought-Focused to Action-Focused

One of the best ways to weaken irrational thoughts is to shift from focusing on them to taking action. Instead of ruminating or debating the thought, do something physical and engaging to redirect your brain's attention:

- Exercise: Go for a walk, stretch, or do something active to reset your mind.
- Engage Your Senses: Listen to music, smell something calming, or focus on an object in front of you.
- Talk to Someone: Shifting to an external conversation helps break internal thought loops.
- Do a Task: Cook, clean, or engage in any small activity that requires focus.

Action interrupts the cycle of irrational thinking, helping you regain control and move forward.

Brain Glitches, Trauma, and Why Cognitive Techniques May Not Work (Yet)

Throughout this chapter, we have discussed strategies such as cognitive defusion, distancing yourself from negative thoughts, and understanding that your thoughts do not define who you are. These tools can significantly reduce the impact of harmful thought patterns, which we call brain glitches. However, if you have found these methods difficult or ineffective, there may be a deeper neurological reason related to unresolved trauma, anxiety, or PTSD.

When trauma remains unresolved, it creates persistent hyperactivity in the amygdala, the part of your brain responsible for detecting threats. This heightened state effectively bypasses your brain's rational control center, the prefrontal cortex, making logical thinking or cognitive distancing extremely difficult (Shin et al., 2006; Rauch et al., 2006). Essentially, your brain is stuck in a fight or flight mode, continually reinforcing negative thought loops or brain glitches, even when you logically recognize they are irrational.

Because of this neurological response, it is critical to first achieve trauma closure before fully benefiting from the cognitive distancing and defusion techniques outlined in this chapter. Trauma closure does not erase past experiences, but it helps your brain turn off the chronic alarm signals, allowing your prefrontal cortex to function effectively once again. Without addressing trauma first, efforts to rationalize or distance yourself emotionally from troubling thoughts may feel frustrating and ineffective (Van der Kolk, 2014; Shapiro, 2017).

In the next chapter, we will delve deeply into the concept of trauma closure, exploring evidence-based approaches that help reset your brain's alarm system. Only after achieving this crucial neurological reset can cognitive strategies fully take hold and support lasting emotional well-being.

A Personal Perspective

There was a time when my irrational thoughts controlled me. I believed that if I had a thought, it must be important, meaningful, and true. But once I learned to step back, zoom out, and distance myself, I realized that my thoughts were just mental noise, not reality.

By treating thoughts as movies to watch, clouds to let pass, or Google Earth images to zoom out from, I stopped giving them so much power. I still experience irrational thoughts like everyone else, but now, instead of fighting them or fearing them, I observe them, detach, and move on. Your thoughts are not you. They are just fleeting mental events. The less you engage with irrational thoughts, the faster they lose their power.

6. Trauma Closure: BioPsycho Therapy (BPT)

The Psychological Cost of Unresolved Trauma: How Lack of Closure Traps the Brain in a Cycle of PTSD and Depression

One of the lesser discussed, yet highly significant contributors to depression and post-traumatic stress disorder (PTSD), is the lack of emotional closure following traumatic experiences. When individuals go through traumatic events, such as abuse, loss, violence, or life-threatening situations, those experiences often remain psychologically "open-ended" if not properly processed. Without closure, the brain tends to enter a persistent loop, constantly revisiting and reinterpreting the traumatic memory in an effort to make sense of it. This neural reactivation is not just psychological; it's biological. Research using neuroimaging has shown that trauma survivors often experience heightened activity in the amygdala (the brain's fear center) and reduced activity in the prefrontal cortex, which is responsible for rational thinking and emotional regulation (Shin et al., 2006).

The failure to achieve closure, whether through emotional resolution, justice, or meaning-making, prevents the traumatic memory from being consolidated and stored like normal memories. Instead, it remains vivid and emotionally charged, leading to flashbacks, nightmares, anxiety, and persistent depressive symptoms. This process is supported by the work of van der Kolk (2014), who demonstrated that traumatic memories are often stored somatically and in fragmented, non-verbal forms, making them difficult to process through standard cognitive means. In his book *The Body Keeps the Score*, he outlines how trauma literally reshapes both brain structure and function, particularly when closure is not achieved.

Moreover, studies suggest that unresolved trauma can lead to a constant state of hyperarousal or hypervigilance, where the nervous system is perpetually on edge, as though the danger is still present. This chronic activation is associated with high levels of cortisol and other stress hormones that contribute to long-term mental health deterioration. A study by Yehuda et al. (1998) found that individuals with PTSD had significantly altered stress hormone regulation, which not only intensified depressive symptoms but also interfered with memory and emotional regulation. These findings confirm that unresolved trauma isn't just "in the past"; it actively disrupts current mental and emotional stability.

While many treatments for depression and PTSD focus on symptom management, addressing the root causes, such as unresolved trauma and lack of closure, is often the key to genuine healing. Without this resolution, the brain remains caught in a feedback loop of fear, stress, and sadness, making long-term recovery difficult without targeted trauma resolution strategies.

Internal vs. External Trauma Closure for PTSD and Emotional Healing

Trauma closure is a vital component of emotional and psychological recovery for individuals suffering from post-traumatic stress disorder (PTSD) and unresolved trauma. Closure may occur through two primary pathways: external closure and internal closure.

External closure involves resolution through outside factors, such as receiving an apology, legal justice, or reconciliation with the perpetrator. While helpful for some, this form of closure is often unrealistic or entirely unavailable in many traumatic circumstances (Herman, 1992).

For example, survivors of childhood abuse, victims of war, or those who experienced trauma from someone who is deceased or unreachable may never have the opportunity for external validation or justice. In these situations, internal closure becomes the only viable path to healing. Without learning how to implement internal closure, individuals are at high risk of chronic emotional distress, including PTSD, depression, and anxiety (Neimeyer, 2000). The inability to find resolution in the absence of external repair can lead to prolonged rumination, emotional dysregulation, and identity disturbances, which are core features of complex trauma (Courtois & Ford, 2009).

Internal closure refers to a self-directed process of healing that includes cognitive reframing, emotional regulation, and narrative restructuring. It allows individuals to assign new meaning to their experiences, reduce the emotional charge associated with the trauma, and separate their identity from the event itself. A key benefit of internal closure is emotional autonomy. Individuals who develop this capacity are no longer dependent on external circumstances or people to feel whole or to move forward. They gain control over their emotional well-being and are able to integrate traumatic experiences into a broader and healthier life narrative. In contrast, those who wait indefinitely for external closure may remain trapped in a cycle of emotional injury and psychological stagnation (Neimeyer, 2000).

Therefore, for many trauma survivors, internal closure is not just beneficial; it is essential. It is the only option in situations where external resolution is impossible or denied. Teaching individuals how to access this internal process is critical to preventing chronic PTSD and promoting lasting recovery.

Gaining a deeper understanding of internal and external trauma closure has profoundly influenced my perspective on overcoming PTSD and emotional trauma. Recognizing that external closure, such as receiving apologies, justice, or validation from others, is often unrealistic or impossible highlighted the critical need for effective methods of internal resolution. Many trauma survivors remain stuck, waiting for external circumstances that may never materialize, leaving them vulnerable to chronic distress and unresolved PTSD symptoms (Herman, 1992; Courtois & Ford, 2009).

Releasing the Past to Heal the Present

One of the greatest barriers to emotional healing is unresolved trauma. When traumatic events occur, whether it's abuse, illness, war, or loss, they can leave behind mental and emotional imprints that distort our view of the world and ourselves. The brain, in its effort to protect us, continues to replay the event, searching for resolution. But without proper closure, we can get stuck in a loop, reliving the past as if it were the present.

Imagine someone who has trained for months to run a marathon. They cross the finish line, but instead of resting or celebrating, they keep looking back, over and over again, checking behind them as if the race never ended. That's what unprocessed trauma does: it keeps your attention locked on the past, draining energy from your present life.

A powerful example of this is when I underwent intensive cancer treatment. Even after surviving, I remained trapped in fear: terrified of the cancer returning, overwhelmed by the possibility of death, and haunted by the memory of the disabling chemo and radiation side effects I had experienced. Though I had healed physically, my brain kept reacting as if I were still in the middle of the battle. This form of trauma, known as medical PTSD, is real and debilitating

(Abbey et al., 2015). The body may be out of danger, but the mind hasn't caught up.

Another example is a soldier returning home from war. Though he is physically in a peaceful environment, his mind continues to replay combat scenes, scanning for danger that no longer exists. Loud noises or crowded places trigger panic because the nervous system is still in survival mode. His body is home, but his brain is still on the battlefield (Van der Kolk, 2015). This is the essence of PTSD: the brain becomes frozen in the past, reacting to old threats as if they are still happening now. Even a smell, a sound, or a thought can trigger a full-blown emotional response, because the memory is stored with all the intensity of the original experience.

Another example is a woman who experienced a traumatic childbirth. Years later, despite having a healthy child, she feels anxious every time she walks into a hospital or hears a baby cry. Her rational mind knows she's safe, but her emotional brain still believes she's in danger. She avoids medical care altogether, not because she's weak, but because her brain never got closure.

Unresolved trauma also creates invisible cages, mental constructs that trap people in cycles of fear and limitation. A person who was bullied in school may grow into an adult who believes they're not worthy of love or success. These beliefs form an emotional prison, but the bars are made of thoughts, not reality. Healing begins when you realize: the cage doesn't exist. The goal of trauma recovery is not to forget, but to bring closure. Closure allows your brain to finally say, "That happened. It's over. I survived." When you stop running from your past and stop looking over your shoulder, you begin to live fully in the now.

Realizing that internal closure provides not only a reliable pathway but often the only practical solution for many individuals, I became inspired to seek and develop therapeutic techniques that facilitate rapid and effective internal healing. Internal closure, which involves personal reprocessing, reframing, and emotional regulation, empowers individuals to find peace independent of external circumstances (Neimeyer, 2000; Thompson et al., 2021). This insight was transformative, motivating me to create and refine BioPsycho Therapy (BPT), a structured, integrative approach that efficiently guides individuals toward rapid internal closure.

My primary goal with BioPsycho Therapy (BPT) was to offer individuals struggling with PTSD and emotional trauma a practical and accessible way to heal internally, without waiting indefinitely for external validation. BPT emphasizes evidence-based cognitive and emotional techniques that promote rapid emotional regulation, cognitive distancing, and personal integration of traumatic experiences.

Illusion of Reality

In psychology, the illusion of reality refers to the brain's tendency to construct a subjective version of the world that may not align with objective truth. This distortion is not a result of imagination or denial, but rather a consequence of automatic cognitive and emotional processes shaped by past experiences, belief systems, and neurobiological responses.

The Brain as an Interpreter, Not a Recorder

The human brain does not passively receive and store reality as it is. Instead, it interprets incoming sensory information through internal filters shaped by emotional states, memory, and prior learning. These mental filters, often referred to as schemas, serve as cognitive shortcuts to help individuals make sense of their environment. However, when influenced by trauma or chronic stress, these filters can become distorted and lead to an inaccurate perception of current circumstances. Neuroscientific research supports this understanding. Studies show that the amygdala, hippocampus, and prefrontal cortex work in concert to interpret experience. In cases of trauma, the amygdala becomes hyperactive while the prefrontal cortex becomes underactive. This imbalance can lead the brain to interpret neutral or safe stimuli as threatening, even in the absence of actual danger (Shin & Liberzon, 2010).

Clinical Examples of Reality Distortion

In individuals with post-traumatic stress disorder (PTSD), reality illusions often manifest as hypervigilance or re-experiencing symptoms. A harmless trigger such as a loud sound may be perceived as life-threatening because the brain is responding to a stored traumatic memory rather than the present environment.

In depression, the illusion often presents as persistent negative beliefs. An individual may internalize thoughts such as "I am worthless" or "Nothing will ever improve" despite having evidence to the contrary. These thoughts are not grounded in current reality but in past emotional injuries or unresolved experiences.

In anxiety disorders, individuals often experience catastrophic thinking. A minor issue, such as a delayed response to a text message or a physical symptom like a headache, may be perceived as a sign of disaster. Although the threat is imagined, the emotional and physiological response is real.

Illusion of Reality: How Trauma Distorts Perception

One of the most important yet misunderstood aspects of anxiety, depression, and PTSD is the brain's relationship with reality. Our perception of the world is not a direct reflection of what is happening around us, but rather an interpretation shaped by our past experiences, beliefs, and emotions. When that interpretation becomes distorted, especially through the lens of trauma, it can create what psychologists refer to as a reality illusion.

A reality illusion occurs when the brain interprets present experiences through outdated or inaccurate mental filters. Instead of seeing things as they are, individuals see them as they fear them to be or as they once were. This illusion often begins after trauma, when the brain encodes an emotionally intense event as a threat and begins to filter future experiences through that unresolved lens. Over time, these distorted interpretations can shape a person's entire worldview, fueling ongoing emotional suffering.

For example, someone who was emotionally abused in childhood may grow into adulthood with the persistent belief, *"I am not good enough,"* even in the face of love and success. That belief is not rooted in current reality. It is a learned emotional truth based on past trauma. Similarly, a person with PTSD might feel sudden panic in a safe environment because their brain misinterprets a sound, smell, or facial expression as a danger signal. Although there is no real threat, the body reacts as if one exists. These are powerful examples of the illusion of reality at work.

In anxiety disorders, this illusion often manifests as catastrophic thinking, believing that something terrible is about to happen despite evidence to the contrary. In depression, it may appear as global negative beliefs such as *"Nothing will ever get better"* or *"I'm worthless."* According to Beck's cognitive theory of depression, these beliefs are part of what are called negative schemas, mental frameworks that were formed in early life and continue to influence perception into adulthood (Beck, 1976). The result is a self-reinforcing cycle. Distorted perceptions lead to emotional pain, which further distorts perception. Neuroscience supports this understanding. Studies using functional MRI have shown that trauma alters activity in key brain regions. The amygdala, which detects threats, becomes overactive, while the prefrontal cortex, responsible for rational thinking and emotional regulation, becomes underactive (Shin & Liberzon, 2010). This imbalance makes it difficult to distinguish between what is real and what is perceived based on past fear.

The danger of the reality illusion is that it feels true. The mind and body respond to imagined threats with the same intensity as real ones. In trauma-informed approaches like BioPsycho Therapy, the goal is to help individuals resolve the root trauma so that the nervous system can stop reacting as if the danger is still happening. Healing begins when individuals realize that thoughts and emotions are not always accurate reflections of reality. The mind can be misled by its own memory systems, especially when those systems have been shaped by trauma.

Why Recognizing the Illusion Matters

Understanding that thoughts and emotions are not always accurate representations of reality is critical for healing. Individuals suffering from anxiety, depression, or PTSD often mistake emotionally charged thoughts for truth. This confusion perpetuates distress and prevents growth. Learning to observe thoughts without immediate judgment or reaction allows individuals to regain cognitive clarity and emotional stability.

Therapeutic interventions that target these illusions are not about ignoring pain but about helping individuals distinguish between what is current and what is remembered, between what is real and what is perceived through a distorted lens. As individuals begin to replace illusion with clarity, they create space for hope, resilience, and lasting change.

The Invisible Cage: How Distorted Thoughts Trap Us

One of the most damaging effects of the reality illusion is the creation of what can be called an invisible cage, a mental prison constructed from distorted, irrational, or emotionally charged thoughts. These thoughts are often so deeply ingrained that they feel real, even when they are completely disconnected from objective reality. The invisible cage is built not with physical barriers but with beliefs, assumptions, and fears that shape how individuals see themselves, others, and the world.

For example, a person struggling with social anxiety may walk into a room and immediately think, *"Everyone is judging me"* or *"They all think I'm awkward."* These thoughts are not based on actual feedback or behavior but are internal projections rooted in past experiences of rejection or embarrassment. Although no one may be paying special attention to them, the brain perceives threat and the body responds with anxiety and tension. The thought feels true, and as a result, the person may avoid social settings altogether, trapped in an invisible cage of imagined criticism.

In depression, this cage often takes the form of hopeless, self-deprecating beliefs. Thoughts like *"I'm broken,"* *"I'll never get better,"* or *"No one could ever love me"* create a sense of emotional paralysis. These beliefs are not the result of current evidence but rather the echo of past trauma, abandonment, or failure. Because the person believes the thought, they behave as if it is true, isolating themselves, refusing help, or giving up on goals they are fully capable of achieving.

People with post-traumatic stress disorder often experience the invisible cage through the lens of safety and control. A combat veteran may believe, *"I can't relax because something bad could happen at any time"* or *"I have to be on guard or I'll be hurt again."* These beliefs are a direct result of the brain's survival mechanisms, which have not updated since the trauma occurred. The threat is no longer present, but the mind and body continue to act as though it is. What makes the invisible cage so powerful is that it is largely unconscious. Most people are not aware that their thoughts are distorted or that they are living inside a cognitive illusion. The bars of the cage are made of thoughts, but those thoughts feel like facts. Without awareness, individuals continue to live inside these cages, not realizing that the door was never locked.

Trauma Closure First: Why Cognitive Tools Won't Work Without It

Many techniques presented in previous chapters, such as cognitive defusion, distancing from negative thoughts, and understanding that your thoughts are not you, are powerful tools for healing. However, these methods often fall short when applied to individuals experiencing unresolved trauma, chronic anxiety, or PTSD. This is because trauma activates a survival mechanism in the brain that overrides logic and rational processing. Specifically, trauma causes hyperactivity in the amygdala, the brain's fear center, while suppressing activity in the prefrontal cortex, which governs reasoning, decision making, and emotional regulation (Shin et al., 2006; Rauch et al., 2000). In simpler terms, you cannot use logic to combat fear when your brain is stuck in survival mode.

This neurological hijack explains why cognitive defusion and distancing techniques don't stick when trauma is unresolved. These strategies require access to the prefrontal cortex, the very region that becomes offline during trauma responses. According to neuroimaging studies, individuals with PTSD show increased amygdala activation and decreased medial prefrontal cortex engagement when exposed to trauma-related stimuli (Rauch et al., 2006). Without first resolving or finding closure for the trauma, attempts at cognitive reappraisal can feel futile or even frustrating. You may intellectually know a thought is irrational yet feel powerless to stop believing it because your emotional brain is still activated.

To deactivate this hypervigilant state, trauma closure is essential. Trauma closure is not about erasing what happened but rather creating a sense of safety, resolution, and meaning around the event. **Only when the amygdala's alarm is turned off can the prefrontal cortex come back online and allow the brain to properly engage in cognitive defusion, mindfulness, and rational distancing.** Without this foundational step, the brain remains in a reactive loop, unable to process or integrate new insights. Understanding this sequence is crucial. If you've struggled with thinking your way out of depression or anxiety, it may not be a failure of mindset. It could be that your nervous system needs closure first. Only then can cognitive strategies begin to take root and guide lasting change.

How BPT Helped Me Overcome PTSD and Depression by Addressing the Root Cause: Unresolved Trauma

My journey to healing from PTSD and depression began with the realization that many traditional treatments were only addressing the symptoms, not the root cause. I had spent years stuck in a cycle of emotional distress, hypervigilance, and hopelessness. Through both personal experience and scientific research, I came to understand that the core issue was unresolved trauma. The memories I hadn't processed, the events I had never found closure for, were replaying in my mind and body again and again. No medication or talk therapy alone could stop that cycle, because they didn't help me complete those past experiences.

This insight led me to develop BPT (BioPsycho Therapy), a new approach that directly targets stored trauma in both the brain and body. I began using a highly powerful magnetic device (MagnaHeal Pro) to stimulate deep tissues and neural pathways while intentionally revisiting the traumatic memories during treatment. The key was not avoiding the trauma but safely bringing it into the session, not to re-traumatize, but to complete the experience. This allowed my nervous system to finally release what it had been holding onto for years.

In just a few sessions, I experienced dramatic changes. For the first time, the traumatic memories no longer had control over me. I was able to process them, find closure, and feel relief that years of conventional treatments couldn't give me. The combination of MagnaHeal Pro stimulation with intentional trauma recall allowed my brain to rewire, release the emotional charge, and return to a calm, balanced state. That is how I overcame both PTSD and depression: not by masking the symptoms, but by confronting and resolving the source.

Today, BPT has become a powerful tool I use with others who are suffering. It's a method born from necessity, experience, and the belief that healing is possible when we treat the whole person, including the mind, body, and nervous system, as one integrated system.

BioPsycho Therapy (BPT): A Breakthrough in Mental Health Treatment

The Birth of BioPsycho Therapy (BPT)

When I first sought help for depression, I was told by therapists that I would need 6–12 months of therapy, with weekly sessions. However, I quickly realized that I did not have the time or financial resources to undergo such an intense and prolonged treatment. At the same time, I had already invented several medical devices, so I asked myself: Is there a way to achieve faster relief from depression without committing to a year of therapy?

I began studying different psychological therapy approaches and discovered that most methods require long-term dedication and consistent effort. The complexity and time-consuming nature of these therapies made me wonder if there was a way to simplify treatment while retaining its effectiveness. This led me to the idea of integrating the most effective therapeutic approaches into a single, streamlined exercise.

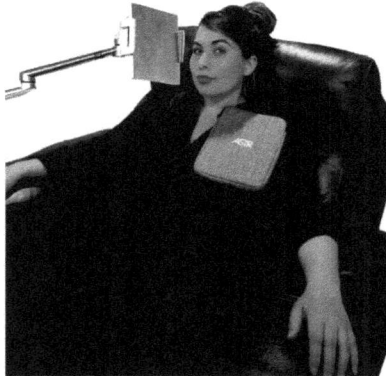

The Role of Magnetic Fields in Mental Health

While researching potential solutions, I stumbled upon an existing method known as Transcranial Magnetic Stimulation (TMS). TMS is a noninvasive procedure that uses magnetic fields to stimulate nerve cells in the brain, helping to improve symptoms of depression. This method works by inducing electric currents in the brain, either eliciting or suppressing action potentials. However, TMS treatment is both expensive and time-consuming; it requires approximately 36 to 40 sessions, with each session lasting 40 minutes over a nine-week period.

Additionally, the cost of a TMS machine is around $56,000, making it inaccessible to many individuals seeking treatment.

At the time, I had already developed a highly powerful magnet designed to reduce inflammation and accelerate the body's healing process. I realized that if magnetic stimulation could influence neural activity, it might be possible to use my magnet, the MagnaHeal Pro, in conjunction with a set of therapeutic exercises that integrate eight different psychological therapy approaches.

The Breakthrough Experiment

Curious about the potential effects, I conducted an experiment on myself. I used MagnaHeal Pro in combination with the therapy exercises that I developed, my stress level was at 9/10 on a scale from 0 to 10 (with 0 being no stress and 10 being severe stress). After completing the session, my stress level dropped to 0 or 1 out of 10, and I experienced an unexpected but profound sense of euphoria throughout the entire day. Initially, I could not believe the results.

To validate my experience, I repeated the treatment multiple times, targeting different psychological stressors, including childhood trauma and anxiety related to my cancer treatment. The results remained consistent. I felt relief from anxiety and depression symptoms, and for the first time, I was able to talk about my traumatic cancer treatment without becoming emotional or breaking into tears. The most astonishing part was that I achieved these results after only a few sessions of BPT. Motivated by these findings, I decided to test this approach on my patients who had psychological trauma, and astonishingly, they reported the same transformative results.

The BioPsycho Therapy (BPT) Approach

BioPsycho Therapy (BPT) is a novel psychotherapeutic approach that integrates noninvasive magnetic fields with psychological therapy techniques. The core principle of BPT is to stimulate nerve cells in the brain responsible for emotional responses, memory recall, and trauma processing while simultaneously executing psychotherapy treatments. The primary focus of BPT is on recalling, desensitizing, and replacing stressful emotions with positive associations.

BPT combines several well-established psychotherapy modalities:

1. **Cognitive Behavioral Therapy (CBT):** Helps identify and restructure negative thought patterns.
2. **Eye Movement Desensitization and Reprocessing (EMDR):** Assists in processing and desensitizing traumatic memories.
3. **Cognitive Defusion**
4. **Rational Emotive Behavior Therapy (REBT)**: Encourages rational thinking to counteract emotional distress.
5. **Psychodynamic Therapy**: Focuses on unconscious influences on behavior.
6. **Positive Psychology:** Enhances well-being through strengths-based interventions.
7. **Trauma-Focused Cognitive Behavioral Therapy (TF-CBT)**
8. **Emotion-Focused Therapy (EFT):** Helps process emotional pain and trauma-related stress.

Magnetic Therapy

Magnetic fields can pass through human tissue without being diminished and without causing harmful effects. This ability to deliver neural stimulation wirelessly makes them an attractive, minimally invasive option for influencing brain activity. Research supports the idea that transcranial magnetic stimulation (TMS) can effectively treat major depressive disorder, particularly in patients who have not responded to conventional antidepressant medication. A systematic review of repetitive transcranial magnetic stimulation (rTMS) for depression concluded that high-quality evidence supports its efficacy in patients who have failed one or fewer medication treatments.

The Impact of Anxiety, Depression, and PTSD on Cardiovascular Health: Understanding the Role of the Amygdala

Anxiety, depression, and post-traumatic stress disorder (PTSD) are often linked to heightened activity in the amygdala, a region of the brain responsible for processing emotional responses, particularly fear and threat. When the amygdala is overactive, especially due to unresolved trauma, it can hijack the brain's normal regulatory functions and initiate a prolonged sympathetic nervous system response. This "fight or flight" activation results in increased blood pressure and heart rate, as the body remains in a state of heightened alert even in the absence of immediate danger. Studies have shown that individuals with chronic anxiety or PTSD often exhibit elevated cardiovascular markers, including resting heart rate and blood pressure, due to this persistent sympathetic dominance (Thayer et al., 2012).

However, when trauma is appropriately processed and resolved through methods such BioPsycho Therapy (BPT), the amygdala's hyperactivity is reduced, allowing the parasympathetic nervous system—the "rest and digest" branch—to regain control. As emotional regulation improves and the brain no longer perceives ongoing threat, physiological signs of relaxation follow. Blood pressure and heart rate begin to decrease, indicating a shift from stress to calm. This physiological response serves as a measurable marker of recovery, showing how emotional healing can directly influence autonomic nervous system balance and cardiovascular health.

Patient Experiences with BPT

In the medical field, practitioners frequently use a numerical rating scale ranging from 0 to 10 to measure a patient's stress level. On this scale, a score of 0 indicates no stress, meaning the patient feels completely calm and relaxed. Conversely, a score of 10 represents extreme or maximal stress, signifying that the patient feels overwhelmed, unable to cope, and intensely distressed. This straightforward numeric system provides clinicians with a reliable, quantifiable way to quickly assess patient stress levels, monitor changes over time, and evaluate the effectiveness of therapeutic interventions (Williamson & Hoggart, 2005).

You can watch live BPT treatment sessions and access documented case studies by scanning the QR code below.

Case Study 1: 20 Years of Depression and PTSD

Previous Failed Treatments: One year of psychotherapy and 12 different antidepressant medications
Stress Level (0–10): 9/10
Before Treatment Vitals: Blood Pressure – 142/70 mmHg, Heart Rate – 58 bpm
Treatment Administered: BioPsycho Therapy (BPT)
After Treatment Vitals: Blood Pressure – 114/59 mmHg, Heart Rate – 56 bpm
Outcome: Stress level reduced to 0/10; depression and PTSD resolved. The patient experienced a feeling of euphoria after the treatment

Case Study 2: Anxiety due to breathing problem - COPD

Stress Level (0–10): 10/10
Before Treatment Vitals: Blood Pressure – 146/107mmHg, Heart Rate – 58 bpm, O2 level 75
Treatment Administered: BioPsycho Therapy (BPT)
After Treatment Vitals: Blood Pressure – 113/71 mmHg, Heart Rate – 75 bpm, O2 level increased to 84 (improved)
Outcome: Stress level reduced to 1-2/10; anxiety resolved.
Follow-up (2 Months): Stress level remained at 0-1/10

Case Study 3: Anxiety & Stress

Stress Level (0–10): 9/10
Before Treatment Vitals: Blood Pressure – 142/95 mmHg, Heart Rate – 109 bpm
Treatment Administered: BioPsycho Therapy (BPT)
After Treatment Vitals: Blood Pressure – 118/78 mmHg, Heart Rate – 79 bpm,
Outcome: Stress level reduced to 0/10,
Follow-up (1 Month): Stress level remained at 0/10

Case Study 4: Anxiety & Depression

Stress Level (0–10): 7/10
Before Treatment Vitals: Blood Pressure – 132/79 mmHg, Heart Rate – 89 bpm
Treatment Administered: BioPsycho Therapy (BPT)

After Treatment Vitals: Blood Pressure – 125/70 mmHg, Heart Rate – 70 bpm,
Outcome: Stress level reduced to 0/10,
Follow-up: Stress level 0/10

Case Study 5: Anxiety

Stress Level (0–10): 7/10
Before Treatment Vitals: Blood Pressure – 122/69 mmHg, Heart Rate – 83 bpm
Treatment Administered: BioPsycho Therapy (BPT)
After Treatment Vitals: Blood Pressure – 104/67 mmHg, Heart Rate – 77 bpm,
Outcome: Stress level reduced to 0/10
Follow-up (1–2 Months): Stress level remained at 0/10

Case Study 6: Anxiety

Stress Level (0–10): 7/10
Before Treatment Vitals: Blood Pressure – 117/74 mmHg, Heart Rate – 74 bpm
Treatment Administered: BioPsycho Therapy (BPT)
After Treatment Vitals: Blood Pressure – 113/74 mmHg, Heart Rate – 68 bpm,
Outcome: Stress level reduced to 0/10

Meditation and the Euphoric Effect with MagnaHeal Pro

Many patients who have undergone BPT describe the euphoric sensation after a session as similar to the "good trip" associated with psychedelic experiences, without hallucinations or loss of consciousness. The treatment provides profound mental clarity, a sense of calm, and an overall mood elevation that lasts well beyond the session itself.

It is very common for patients to experience a euphoric effect when combining meditation with MagnaHeal Pro therapy. As the device promotes deep tissue relaxation and nervous system balance, the body naturally shifts into a state of safety and calm. This creates the ideal environment for meditation to produce a powerful release, often felt as a wave of emotional lightness, peace, or even joy. Many patients describe feeling as though a weight has been lifted, allowing them to access a deeper sense of clarity and closure. This euphoric state supports trauma healing by calming the mind, reducing physical tension, and enhancing emotional processing.

Scaling BPT for Wider Accessibility

Once I observed consistent results across different patients, I developed a certification program for healthcare providers to integrate BPT into their practice. This course equips professionals with the knowledge and tools to administer BPT effectively. Additionally, I created a program for individuals to implement BPT at home, ensuring that anyone struggling with psychological distress could benefit from this innovative treatment without requiring prolonged and expensive therapy sessions.

Path to Trauma Closure

Trauma isn't just stored in the mind; it lives in the body, influencing how we think, feel, and respond to everyday experiences. BPT recognizes the interconnectedness of the body, mind, and environment. It combines magnetic therapy with emotional processing, behavioral change, and somatic awareness to help release trauma from the places where it has been physically and neurologically stored.

Trauma closure begins with awareness. We gently explore how the body reacts to stress, how the mind processes past pain, and how behavior patterns may have developed as survival mechanisms. Through hands-on techniques, and guided cognitive distancing, BPT helps patients safely reconnect with their bodies and reprocess trauma without reliving it.

The goal is not to erase the past, but to integrate it, freeing the body from chronic tension and the mind from loops of fear, guilt, or shame. When the nervous system learns safety again, healing follows. This is trauma closure: not forgetting, but no longer suffering.

Conclusion

True healing from PTSD and depression often requires more than symptom management; it requires addressing unresolved trauma at its root. For many, the pain of the past is not just a memory; it lives in the body and mind as if it is still happening. When external closure is not possible, when no apology is given, justice is denied, or reconciliation never comes, internal closure becomes not just important but essential.

Internal closure is the process of completing unresolved experiences from within. It allows the brain and nervous system to stop replaying traumatic events, freeing the mind from loops of fear, shame, or guilt. By acknowledging what happened, processing the emotions, and reframing the meaning, individuals can reclaim their personal power and shift from victimhood to healing. It does not mean forgetting the trauma; it means integrating it into your life story without letting it define your future.

This shift is what enables long-term emotional recovery. When trauma is no longer open-ended, the nervous system learns to feel safe again. The body relaxes. The mind quiets. And for the first time, many people feel a deep sense of relief, not because the past changed, but because their relationship to it did. This is what makes internal closure such a vital piece of depression recovery: it ends the cycle of emotional reactivation and creates space for peace, clarity, and resilience.

BioPsycho Therapy (BPT) represents a revolutionary approach to mental health treatment by combining powerful psychological therapies with the noninvasive effects of magnetic fields. By simplifying treatment and significantly reducing the time required for symptom relief, BPT challenges the conventional notion that long-term therapy is the only path to healing. This method not only provides rapid and lasting results but also empowers both healthcare providers and individuals to take control of their mental well-being in a cost-effective and accessible manner.

7. The Illusion of Control

At some point, nearly everyone has caught themselves trying to influence the uncontrollable. A sports fan might insist on wearing a "lucky" jersey to help their team win, genuinely believing it will sway the outcome (The Decision Lab, n.d.). You may have pressed an elevator's "close door" button repeatedly, half-suspecting it does nothing, yet feeling better for having done something. These are everyday examples of the illusion of control, our tendency to overestimate our ability to control external events. In reality, we often have far less control over outcomes than we imagine, but our minds frequently trick us into feeling otherwise (The Decision Lab, n.d.).

This chapter explores the science behind the illusion of control, why we cling to it, and how it affects our decisions, mental health, and relationships. It also offers practical insights on accepting what we cannot control and focusing on what we can, such as our own actions, mindset, and responses.

What Is the Illusion of Control?

The illusion of control is a cognitive bias in which people believe they have influence over outcomes that are actually determined by chance or external forces (The Decision Lab, n.d.; Wikipedia, 2023). Psychologist Ellen Langer first identified this bias in 1975, observing that people often behave as if random events are subject to their will. This phenomenon is considered one of the "positive illusions" in psychology, alongside unrealistic optimism and illusory superiority. These biases create a rosier perception of our control and abilities than objective reality justifies. Even when outcomes are purely random or governed by external factors, the illusion of control leads us to believe, *"I can make a difference."*

For example, someone might feel safer on an airplane if they perform a personal good-luck ritual, as if it prevents accidents. In one experiment, college students undergoing virtual reality therapy for fear of heights were told they could control a simulated elevator, when in fact, some could not. Interestingly, those who were falsely told they had control reported feeling just as much in control as participants who actually did, simply because they believed they were in charge (Wikipedia, 2023).

This demonstrates how our perception of control can override reality. Since we lack direct insight into actual control, we rely on feelings and cues, which can be misleading. Everyday examples of the illusion of control include:

- Gambling and Lotteries: People often believe they can influence luck. A classic study showed that participants who chose their own lottery numbers were far more reluctant to trade their ticket for another, even when offered one with better odds of winning (Wikipedia, 2023). Similarly, gamblers at a dice table might throw the dice harder hoping for higher numbers or softer for lower numbers, even though the odds remain the same (Clearer Thinking, n.d.).
- Superstitions and Rituals: Many people carry a lucky charm into a job interview or arrange their desk a certain way before an exam, believing these actions will increase their chances of success (The Decision Lab, n.d.).
- Placebo Buttons: Many crosswalk buttons and elevator close-door buttons do nothing, yet people press them believing they speed up the process (Psychological Science, n.d.). These placebo buttons exist to make people feel they have control, even when they don't.

These examples illustrate how the illusion of control provides comfort by reducing uncertainty and anxiety.

How the Illusion of Control Affects Mental Health

The illusion of control has a two-sided impact on mental health. On one hand, a sense of control can be beneficial, fostering motivation and resilience. On the other, clinging to unrealistic control beliefs can lead to stress, anxiety, and frustration.

1. Positive Effects: Studies show that non-depressed individuals tend to have mildly inflated perceptions of control, which helps them remain optimistic and persistent (Wikipedia, 2023).
2. Anxiety and Stress: People who try to control everything, from relationships to external events, often experience high levels of stress. When their expectations don't match reality, they may feel overwhelmed and anxious (Clearer Thinking, n.d.).

3. Self-Blame and Guilt: When people assume too much responsibility for outcomes, they may blame themselves for failures beyond their control, leading to unnecessary guilt (The Decision Lab, n.d.).
4. Learned Helplessness: In contrast, some people experience learned helplessness, where they give up control altogether, believing their actions make no difference (Wikipedia, 2023).

Balancing realistic control and acceptance is key to maintaining mental well-being.

The illusion of control is a deeply ingrained psychological bias that tricks us into overestimating our influence over external events. While it can boost confidence and motivation, it can also lead to frustration, stress, and poor decision-making. Recognizing when we truly have control and when we do not allows us to focus on what we can change: our own actions, mindset, and responses, while letting go of unrealistic expectations. By shifting our focus to what we can influence, we can cultivate greater peace of mind, healthier relationships, and improved well-being.

The Illusion of Control: Letting Go and Focusing on What You Can Change

For years, I struggled with the illusion of control, believing that if I tried hard enough, I could control people, situations, or outcomes. I would overthink conversations, anticipate every possible reaction, and convince myself that my efforts could influence circumstances far beyond my reach. But no matter how much I planned, worried, or strategized, life had its own way of unfolding. The truth is, the only thing we truly control is our own actions and responses, not other people, not their decisions, and certainly not every outcome.

Recognizing this has been one of the most liberating realizations of my life. When we cling to the illusion of control, we set ourselves up for disappointment, stress, and frustration. But when we learn to let go of what we cannot change, we free ourselves from unnecessary anxiety and focus on what truly matters: our own growth, mindset, and choices.

Why Do We Believe We Have Control?

The illusion of control is a cognitive bias, a mental shortcut that makes us believe we have more influence over events than we actually do. Psychologists have studied this phenomenon for decades, showing that humans naturally overestimate their ability to shape outcomes, even in situations driven by chance (Langer, 1975).

There are several reasons why our minds convince us that we have control when we do not:

1. We Want Predictability: The brain craves certainty because it makes us feel safe. When things feel unpredictable, we try to create a sense of control, even if it's an illusion.
2. We Mistake Influence for Control: Just because our actions impact a situation does not mean we fully control the outcome. Influence is not the same as control.
3. We Link Effort to Success: We often believe that if we try harder, we can control everything, but some factors are beyond our reach, no matter how much effort we put in.

This illusion can be comforting in the short term, but in reality, it often leads to frustration, anxiety, and exhaustion.

The Only Thing You Control: Your Actions

The hard truth is that we cannot control:
- Other people's thoughts, feelings, or actions
- Unexpected life events
- The opinions of others
- How people respond to us
- Every outcome, no matter how well we plan

But we can control:
- How we react to situations
- Our attitude and mindset
- The choices we make
- The effort we put into our own growth
- How we manage our emotions

Real peace comes from shifting our focus from what we can't control to what we can.

Practical Ways to Let Go of the Illusion of Control

1. Watch Life Like a Movie

Imagine you are in a movie theater, watching life unfold on the screen. Instead of trying to control the plot, imagine you are simply an observer. You can react, make choices, and adapt, but you can't rewrite the script.

When faced with a frustrating situation, ask yourself:
- *"Am I the director of this movie, or just a character experiencing it?"*
- *"Is this something I can actually control, or just something I need to respond to?"*

This shift in perspective can reduce stress and help you detach from the need to control everything.

2. Ask Yourself: Is This Mine to Control?

Whenever you feel anxious or frustrated about a situation, pause and ask:

- *"Is this within my control?"*
- *"If I let go of this worry, would I be freer?"*
- *"What action can I take instead of trying to control this?"*

By focusing only on what is actually within your power, you avoid unnecessary stress.

3. Don't Pick Up Other People's Problems

Many of us try to fix others, whether it's a friend struggling, a partner making bad choices, or a colleague stressing out. But we can't control other people's lives. Instead of absorbing other people's emotions, remind yourself:

- *"This is their experience, not mine."*

- *"I can support them, but I can't fix it for them."*
- *"The best way to help is to focus on being the best version of myself."*

4.Picture a Tug-of-War Rope, Then Drop It

Trying to control a situation is like pulling on a rope in a tug-of-war battle. The harder you pull, the more resistance you face. The tension grows, the frustration builds. But the moment you drop the rope, the struggle stops. Next time you find yourself mentally wrestling with something you can't control, visualize yourself dropping the rope and walking away.

5. Replace "Why Is This Happening?" with "What Can I Do?"

When things don't go as planned, it's easy to get stuck asking:

- *"Why is this happening?"*
- *"Why won't they change?"*
- *"Why can't I make this work?"*

These questions keep you stuck in frustration and resistance. Instead, shift to action-based thinking:

- *"What can I do right now?"*
- *"How can I adapt?"*
- *"What lesson can I learn from this?"*

Focusing on solutions instead of problems helps you regain a sense of calm and control over your own actions.

6. Destroyed by the Wave or Ride the Wave

In reality, trying to control the uncontrollable often creates more suffering. Life, like the ocean, brings waves that are beyond our control: loss, change, illness, disappointment. When we try to stand rigid against these waves, they knock us down. But when we adopt a posture of flexibility through acceptance, adaptation, and resilience, we learn to move with the current rather than against it. True strength lies in recognizing what we cannot control and focusing our energy on what we can, including our actions, our mindset, and our response.

You Have Control

One of the most exhausting aspects of depression is the sense of helplessness it brings: the feeling that life is happening to you and that there's little you can do to change it. Often, people struggling with depression try to regain a sense of control by fixating on things outside of their influence, such as other people's actions, the past, or unpredictable life events. This illusion of control creates even more stress, disappointment, and emotional pain, because these areas can't be managed, no matter how much we try. The key to emotional freedom is not in controlling the uncontrollable, but in reclaiming control where it actually exists: within your own daily choices and actions.

You may not be able to control what has happened to you or how others behave, but you *do* have control over how you care for your body, your mind, and your environment. This chapter invites you to redirect your energy toward what you can influence by implementing the 14 elements outlined in this book.

You can choose to nourish your body with healing foods. You can correct vitamin and hormone imbalances. You can set boundaries with screen time, declutter your space, and engage in practices like mindfulness, forgiveness, and behavior change. These are not small acts; they are powerful decisions that send a message to your brain and body: *I am showing up for my healing.*

By letting go of the illusion that you must control everything and focusing instead on these actionable steps, you shift from passive suffering to active recovery. Healing is not about forcing the world to conform to your expectations; it's about transforming the way you respond to the world. Each of the 14 tools in this book gives you a place to start, a way to participate in your own healing journey. Depression thrives in passivity, but hope grows when you begin to take ownership of your internal and external environment. Ultimately, it's not about controlling every outcome; it's about realizing that you already possess the ability to influence your health, mindset, and environment. When you reclaim this kind of control, rooted in self-care and grounded action, the illusion fades, and what's left is true empowerment.

A Personal Perspective

There was a time when I tried to control everything: the way people saw me, the way situations unfolded, even the way people reacted to me. If something went wrong, I would immediately think, *"What did I do wrong?"* or *"How can I fix this?"* The more I tried to control the uncontrollable, the more stressed and exhausted I became.

It wasn't until I truly accepted that I only control my own actions that I started feeling free. I stopped trying to force outcomes, change people, or predict every detail of life. Instead, I started focusing on what I could do:

✔ Taking care of my health
✔ Setting boundaries with toxic people
✔ Letting go of relationships that drained me
✔ Accepting that some things are beyond my control
✔ Trusting that I will adapt, no matter what happens

Letting go of the illusion of control does not mean giving up; it means shifting your energy to what actually matters. When you release the need to control everything, you gain something even more valuable: peace.

Final Thought: What You Can Control, What You Can't

⬛ What You CAN Control:
☑ Your actions
☑ Your words
☑ Your effort
☑ Your mindset
☑ Implementing the 14 practical tips from this book

✖ What You CANNOT Control:
🚫 Other people's reactions
🚫 Life's unpredictable events

🚫 The past
🚫 Every outcome

By focusing on what you can change, you free yourself from the stress of trying to control the uncontrollable. Life becomes lighter, easier, and more fulfilling.

8. Change is the Only Constant

Life is defined by its constant state of change. From birth to death, our journey is marked by continuous transitions. Embracing change as an inevitable part of life helps us navigate both joy and adversity more effectively. As the Greek philosopher Heraclitus famously said, "The only constant in life is change."

Understanding the Nature of Change

Life unfolds in seasons, each with its purpose. Ecclesiastes 3:1-2 beautifully encapsulates this truth: "To everything there is a season, and a time to every purpose under the heaven: a time to be born, and a time to die." This scripture illustrates life's inherent cycles: times of happiness and sorrow, growth and loss, beginnings and endings.

The Importance of Flexibility

When we resist change, we become vulnerable to emotional distress and mental strain. Studies consistently highlight that adaptability is critical for mental health. Research by Kashdan and Rottenberg (2010) found that psychological flexibility significantly improves emotional resilience, reduces anxiety, and enhances overall well-being. Another study by Hayes et al. (2012) demonstrated that individuals who adapt flexibly to life's inevitable changes report higher levels of satisfaction and lower levels of depression.

Like ocean waves, life's changes come relentlessly. We can choose either to ride the waves gracefully or to resist and risk being crushed by them. Recognizing the transient nature of all experiences empowers us to move through life with wisdom and strength.

Crushed by the Wave: Resistance to Change

When life takes an unexpected turn, some people cling tightly to the way things used to be. They resist change, replay old routines, and struggle to accept new possibilities. This resistance often leads to frustration, anxiety, and eventually emotional exhaustion. The harder they try to hold on to control, the more overwhelmed they become. Rather than adjusting to the new reality, they become stuck in a cycle of regret and hopelessness. The wave of change doesn't pass; it crashes.

Riding the Wave: Adapting and Accepting Change

Others respond to change with flexibility. Even when faced with loss or uncertainty, they allow themselves to feel and process the shift. Instead of fighting the current, they look for new rhythms, seek support, and explore different paths forward. Acceptance doesn't mean liking the change; it means choosing to move with it rather than against it. In doing so, they often discover unexpected strength, resilience, and peace. The wave still comes, but instead of being crushed by it, they learn to ride it.

Change Is the Norm

Just as we naturally adapt to different climates by putting on warmer clothes in winter and lighter clothes in summer, we must also adapt emotionally and mentally to life's changes. Resistance to the cold won't stop winter from coming; similarly, resisting life's changes won't stop them from happening. Instead, learning to adapt smoothly helps us thrive regardless of circumstances.

Practical Steps to Embrace Change

1. **Acknowledge and Accept:** Recognize and accept that change is inevitable and universal. Acceptance is the first step toward adapting effectively.
2. **Practice Mindfulness:** Regular mindfulness meditation increases emotional resilience, helping us remain calm and centered during times of transition (Shapiro et al., 2006).
3. **Build Support Networks:** Maintain strong connections with friends, family, or support groups. Social connections offer valuable emotional support during periods of significant change.
4. **Maintain Perspective:** Remind yourself that difficult moments are temporary. Reflecting on past experiences of overcoming change can reinforce confidence in your resilience.
5. **Set Realistic Expectations:** Be patient with yourself and others during transitions. Allow time for adaptation and growth.
6. **Stay Flexible:** Cultivate mental flexibility by continuously learning and seeking new experiences. Flexibility enables quicker adaptation to life's inevitable changes

Conclusion

Change is not only inevitable; it is essential. Our ability to remain flexible and resilient determines our emotional health and life satisfaction. Rather than resisting the waves of change and being crushed, choose to ride them with confidence and grace, knowing each wave, however fierce, will eventually pass. Embrace change as your ally, guiding you to continuous growth and deeper fulfillment.

9. Forgiveness

Healing Through Forgiveness

Depression is often deeply intertwined with unresolved emotions such as anger, resentment, and guilt. Forgiveness toward others and oneself can significantly reduce these emotional burdens, promoting emotional resilience and overall mental wellness.

Understanding Forgiveness

Forgiveness involves a conscious decision to let go of resentment or vengeance toward individuals who have caused you harm, regardless of whether their actions were justified or not. It's essential to recognize that forgiveness does not equate to forgetting, condoning, or excusing harmful behaviors. Rather, it frees you from the negative emotions that hinder your mental and emotional health.

The Science Behind Forgiveness and Depression

Multiple studies have documented forgiveness's profound impact on emotional and physical health. Research by Toussaint et al. (2016) revealed significant reductions in depressive symptoms, anxiety, and stress following forgiveness therapy. Another prominent study by Wade, Hoyt, Kidwell, and Worthington (2014) demonstrated that forgiveness interventions significantly reduced depression, increased emotional resilience, and promoted overall psychological well-being. Furthermore, a meta-analysis by Akhtar and Barlow (2018) confirmed that forgiveness therapy improves emotional regulation, reduces depressive symptoms, and enhances overall life satisfaction.

Forgiveness is deeply rooted in biblical teaching. Scripture emphasizes forgiveness as both a spiritual duty and a path toward personal peace. In Matthew 6:14-15, it is stated: "For if you forgive others their trespasses, your heavenly Father will also forgive you. But if you do not forgive others their trespasses, neither will your Father forgive your trespasses." This highlights forgiveness as essential to spiritual and emotional healing.

Similarly, Colossians 3:13 advises, "Bear with each other and forgive one another if any of you has a grievance against someone. Forgive as the Lord forgave you." This principle encourages individuals to reflect divine forgiveness in their personal relationships, fostering harmony and emotional freedom.

Benefits of Forgiveness

Forgiveness provides numerous mental, emotional, and physical benefits, including:
- Reduced stress and anxiety
- Lower risk of depression recurrence
- Improved emotional well-being and resilience
- Enhanced relationships and interpersonal trust
- Better cardiovascular health and lower blood pressure
- Improved immune function
- Increased self-esteem and self-worth

Practical Steps to Implement Forgiveness

1. Recognize and Acknowledge the Hurt: Clearly identify and validate your feelings. Journaling or reflective writing can clarify your emotions and facilitate emotional processing.

2. Make a Conscious Decision to Forgive: Understand forgiveness as a personal choice aimed at improving your mental health. Clearly declare your intention to forgive as a proactive step toward healing.

3. Cultivate Empathy: Attempt to understand the perspective and context of the person who harmed you. Empathy can diminish feelings of resentment and promote emotional healing.

4. Practice Mindfulness and Compassion: Engage in regular mindfulness meditation to cultivate self-awareness and compassion. Studies, such as those by Fredrickson et al. (2008), have demonstrated that mindfulness practices enhance emotional regulation and resilience.

5. Communicate and Seek Closure (If Appropriate): Where possible and safe, communicate your feelings to the person involved to achieve closure. Alternatively, writing unsent letters detailing your feelings can provide therapeutic relief.

Forgiving Yourself

9. Forgiveness

Self-forgiveness is crucial in overcoming depression, as self-blame and guilt often perpetuate depressive cycles. Research by Hall and Fincham (2005) highlights the critical role of self-forgiveness in reducing depressive symptoms and promoting mental health. Practicing self-forgiveness means accepting personal shortcomings, understanding everyone makes mistakes, and actively releasing self-directed negative emotions.

Conclusion

Forgiveness is a transformative practice that empowers individuals to overcome depression by addressing and releasing deep-seated negative emotions. Embracing forgiveness as a regular practice enables sustained emotional freedom, fosters resilience, and significantly enhances overall mental and physical health. Begin your journey toward healing today by integrating forgiveness into your daily life.

10. Limit Screen Time

The Impact of Screen Time and Social Media on Mental Health

For years, I struggled with overuse of screens and social media, often losing hours scrolling through feeds, consuming endless information, and feeling mentally drained. It wasn't until I began studying the effects of screen time on mental health that I realized the toll it was taking. Research shows that excessive screen use, especially prolonged exposure to social media and smartphones, can contribute to anxiety, depression, sleep disturbances, and reduced attention span (Twenge et al., 2018).

Today, screens are an inescapable part of daily life. We rely on them for work, education, and entertainment. However, when screen time becomes excessive, it disrupts mental well-being, increases stress, and diminishes real-life social connections. This chapter explores the research on how screens and social media affect mental health, why they contribute to depression and anxiety, and provides practical strategies to set healthy screen time limits.

The Link Between Screen Time and Mental Health

Numerous studies have linked excessive screen time, particularly on social media, to increased rates of depression, anxiety, and stress.

1. **Depression and Social Media Use**
   Research has shown that higher social media use is strongly associated with increased depression and anxiety, especially among adolescents and young adults (Keles et al., 2020). A study by Twenge et al. (2018) found that teenagers who spend **more than three hours per day** on social media are at a higher risk for mental health issues, including self-harm and suicidal thoughts. The constant exposure to curated, unrealistic portrayals of life on social media can lead to poor self-esteem, body dissatisfaction, and increased feelings of loneliness.
2. **The Dopamine Loop and Addiction**
   Social media platforms are designed to be addictive by exploiting the brain's dopamine reward system, the same system activated by gambling and drug use (Montag et al., 2019). Each notification, like, or comment triggers a dopamine release, making people crave more engagement. This cycle keeps

users hooked, leading to compulsive checking and difficulty disengaging, which contributes to stress and sleep disturbances.

3. **Screen Time and Sleep Disruptions**
The blue light emitted from screens suppresses melatonin production, the hormone responsible for sleep regulation (Chang et al., 2015). Studies indicate that using screens before bed leads to delayed sleep onset, poor sleep quality, and increased fatigue. Lack of sleep is a major risk factor for depression and anxiety (Leone & Sigman, 2020).

4. **Reduced Attention Span and Cognitive Overload**
Excessive screen use fragments attention and reduces the brain's ability to focus deeply (Carr, 2011). Research shows that constant exposure to fast-paced digital content decreases sustained attention, making it harder to concentrate on tasks like reading, problem-solving, and critical thinking (Wilmer et al., 2017). Over time, this contributes to cognitive fatigue, stress, and decreased productivity.

How Social Media Fuels Anxiety and Depression

1. Comparison and Unrealistic Expectations

Social media platforms encourage constant comparison. People see filtered, edited, and staged versions of others' lives, which can create a false perception of reality. This can lead to:
- Feeling inadequate when comparing oneself to others (Fardouly et al., 2015).
- Increased body dissatisfaction due to unrealistic beauty standards (Perloff, 2014).
- Higher rates of depression and anxiety from negative self-evaluation (Twenge et al., 2018).

2. Fear of Missing Out (FOMO) and Social Anxiety

Social media creates a fear of missing out (FOMO), the feeling that others are enjoying life more than you. Research shows that FOMO contributes to anxiety, low self-worth, and compulsive social media checking (Elhai et al., 2018).

3. Online Harassment and Cyberbullying

Prolonged exposure to negative online interactions, such as cyberbullying, hate speech, or criticism, increases stress and can lead to depressive symptoms (Keles et al., 2020). Unlike in-person bullying, cyberbullying follows victims everywhere, making it harder to escape.

4. Social Media and Loneliness

Although social media is designed to connect people, excessive use can actually lead to social isolation. A study found that individuals who spent more than two hours daily on social media were twice as likely to feel lonely compared to those who used it sparingly (Primack et al., 2017).

Smart Watch

I intentionally limit my Apple Watch use to work hours and avoid wearing it at home or on weekends to reduce screen time and minimize stress. By doing so, I create a clear boundary between my professional and personal life, allowing myself to disconnect from constant notifications and digital distractions.

Research suggests that continuous exposure to screens can lead to increased stress, anxiety, and cognitive overload (Mark et al., 2017). By removing the watch outside of work, I reduce the psychological burden of being constantly "on" and give my mind the space to relax and recharge. This practice aligns with digital detox strategies, which emphasize intentional technology use to improve focus, productivity, and overall mental clarity (Ward et al., 2017). Over time, I have noticed improved sleep, better work-life balance, and a greater sense of control over my daily routine. This conscious approach helps me stay present in my personal life while maintaining efficiency at work.

News & Stock Markets

Constantly consuming news and monitoring stock markets can have significant physiological and psychological effects, often contributing to chronic stress and anxiety. The human brain is naturally wired to focus on threats, a survival mechanism known as the negativity bias (Rozin & Royzman, 2001). News channels capitalize on this by emphasizing negative or sensationalized stories, as fear-driven content increases viewer engagement and boosts profits through higher ratings and advertising revenue (Soroka et al., 2019). However, this exposure to distressing news triggers the body's stress response, increasing cortisol levels, elevating heart rate, and reinforcing a cycle of anxiety and hypervigilance (McEwen, 2007).

Similarly, frequently checking stock market fluctuations can activate the same stress pathways, leading to heightened emotional volatility and decision fatigue (Frydman & Camerer, 2016). Since individuals have no control over global events or daily market changes, excessive monitoring leads to a sense of helplessness, exacerbating stress-related conditions such as insomnia, high blood pressure, and burnout. Limiting news and stock updates to designated times or focusing only on long-term trends rather than daily fluctuations can help mitigate these effects, promoting better mental clarity and overall well-being.

Practical Strategies to Limit Screen Time and Improve Mental Health

1. Set Daily Screen Limits
   - Use screen time tracking apps to monitor daily usage.
   - Set a daily screen time limit (e.g., one hour on social media).
   - Designate screen-free hours, especially in the morning and before bed.
2. Reduce Social Media Addiction
   - Turn off notifications to avoid compulsive checking.
   - Unfollow accounts that make you feel negative or self-conscious.
   - Use "Do Not Disturb" mode to stay focused and present.
   - Schedule one or two designated times per day to check social media.
3. Improve Sleep Hygiene
   - Avoid screens at least one hour before bed.
   - Use blue light filters or night mode on devices.
   - Replace nighttime screen time with reading, journaling, or relaxation techniques.
4. Prioritize Face-to-Face Interaction
   - Make a habit of meeting friends and family in person rather than relying on virtual interactions.
   - Join social groups, clubs, or activities to build real-life connections.
5. Create Screen-Free Spaces
   - Designate the bedroom and dining areas as screen-free zones.
   - Keep phones away from the dinner table to encourage conversation.

6. Replace Screen Time with Healthy Activities
  • Swap social media scrolling with exercise, meditation, or outdoor activities.
  • Take frequent breaks from screens throughout the day.
  • Engage in hobbies like reading, painting, or playing an instrument.
7. Digital Detox: Try a Social Media Break
  • Start with a one-day digital detox, then gradually extend it.
  • Temporarily delete social media apps or use features that limit scrolling.
  • Set up "No Social Media Weekends" or screen-free evenings.

Conclusion

While technology and social media are valuable tools, excessive screen time can negatively impact mental health. Studies show a strong connection between social media use and increased depression, anxiety, and sleep disturbances. However, by setting limits, prioritizing real-life connections, and practicing mindful screen use, we can regain control over our mental well-being.
If you find yourself constantly glued to a screen, start small: limit usage, take digital detoxes, and focus on real-world experiences. The goal isn't to eliminate screens entirely, but to create a healthier balance that enhances life, rather than consuming it.

11. Declutter Your Home

Declutter Your House: The Mental Health Benefits of a Tidy Space

For years, I struggled with clutter. My home was filled with unused items, piles of paperwork, and disorganized spaces, and I didn't realize how much it was affecting my mental health. Every time I walked into a messy room, I felt overwhelmed, anxious, and mentally exhausted. But once I began decluttering, I noticed a significant shift in my mood, focus, and overall well-being.

Research supports the connection between clutter and mental health, showing that excessive mess contributes to stress, anxiety, and even depression (Ferrari et al., 2018). In contrast, a clean, organized space has been linked to improved focus, better sleep, and reduced stress levels (Saxbe & Repetti, 2010). This chapter explores how clutter impacts mental health, the science behind decluttering and well-being, and practical strategies to create a tidy, stress-free environment.

How Clutter Affects Mental Health

Clutter is more than just an eyesore; it can have serious psychological effects. Studies suggest that living in a cluttered environment can contribute to chronic stress, anxiety, cognitive overload, and even depression.

1. **Clutter Increases Stress and Anxiety**
   Research shows that cluttered spaces increase cortisol levels, the body's primary stress hormone (Saxbe & Repetti, 2010). A study on working parents found that mothers who described their homes as "cluttered" or "messy" had significantly higher cortisol levels throughout the day compared to those with more organized homes. This suggests that visual chaos contributes to ongoing stress, making it harder to relax at home. High cortisol levels are associated with anxiety, irritability, and difficulty concentrating (Saxbe & Repetti, 2010).

2. **Clutter and Depression**
   A study on hoarding disorder found that excessive accumulation of possessions is linked to increased depressive symptoms (Frost et al., 2012). While hoarding is an extreme example, even moderate clutter can contribute to low energy, feelings of hopelessness, and difficulty making decisions.

Another study found that people who struggle with clutter often experience higher levels of procrastination, avoidance behaviors, and emotional distress (Ferrari et al., 2018).

3. **Clutter Overloads the Brain**
   The human brain is not wired to handle excessive visual stimuli. Neuroscience research indicates that clutter competes for our cognitive resources, reducing the brain's ability to focus and process information efficiently (McMains & Kastner, 2011).

4. **Clutter and Poor Sleep Quality**
   A study published in *Sleep* found that people who sleep in cluttered bedrooms are more likely to experience sleep disturbances and insomnia (Timpano et al., 2017). Messy environments trigger subconscious stress, making it harder for the brain to relax before bedtime. Researchers suggest that tidying up before sleep may improve sleep quality and mental relaxation.

5. When surrounded by clutter, the brain struggles to filter out distractions, leading to:
   1. Decreased productivity
   2. Shorter attention span
   3. Increased feelings of overwhelm

6. A cluttered workspace can significantly hinder concentration and efficiency. (Rosenbaum et al., 2014).

The Psychological Benefits of Decluttering

Decluttering is not just about cleaning; it's a mental reset. Research shows that an organized environment is associated with lower stress, improved focus, and enhanced emotional well-being.

1. **A Clean Space Reduces Stress:** Studies confirm that people who maintain cleaner homes report lower stress levels (Saxbe & Repetti, 2010). Decluttering gives a sense of control and order, reducing the chaos that fuels anxiety.

2. **Decluttering Boosts Productivity:** An organized workspace allows for better concentration and efficiency. Research shows that people working in minimalist environments perform tasks faster and with fewer errors compared to those in cluttered spaces (McMains & Kastner, 2011).
3. **Improves Mood and Emotional Well-Being:** A study on the effects of home organization found that people who declutter experience an increase in positive emotions and reduced depressive symptoms (Ferrari et al., 2018). The act of decluttering provides a sense of achievement and control, leading to better mental clarity and emotional stability.
4. **Encourages Mindfulness and Letting Go:** Decluttering forces us to make intentional choices about what we keep and what we discard. This process fosters mindfulness, helping us let go of emotional attachments to unnecessary objects (Cherrier et al., 2010).

Practical Strategies to Declutter Your Home

Decluttering doesn't have to be overwhelming. Here are practical steps to simplify the process and create a clutter-free environment:

1. Start Small: One Area at a Time
   - Begin with a single drawer, closet, or room instead of trying to declutter your entire home at once.
   - Focus on one category (e.g., clothes, papers, or kitchen items) before moving on to the next.
2. The 5-Second Rule: Quick Decision-Making
   - Pick up an item and ask yourself in five seconds: *Do I use it? Do I love it?* If not, let it go.
   - Avoid overthinking; trust your first instinct.
3. The 90/90 Rule (Minimalist Approach)
   - Ask yourself: *Have I used this item in the last 90 days? Will I use it in the next 90 days?*
   - If the answer is no, donate, recycle, or discard it.
4. Declutter by Categories, Not Rooms
   - Organizing expert Marie Kondo suggests decluttering by categories instead of rooms (Kondo, 2014).
   - Example: Sort through all clothes first, then move to books, kitchenware, sentimental items, etc.

5. The One-Year Rule
   - If you haven't worn, used, or needed an item in over a year, it's time to let it go.
   - Exception: Seasonal items (e.g., holiday decorations, winter coats).
6. Create a Decluttering Routine
   - Set aside 10-15 minutes daily to maintain organization.
   - Designate one day per month for a deep declutter session.
7. Digital Decluttering
   - Unsubscribe from unread emails and notifications.
   - Delete unused apps and files from your phone and computer.
   - Organize digital photos and documents to reduce clutter.

The Emotional Side of Letting Go

Decluttering isn't just about cleaning; it's about emotional release. Many people hold onto items due to sentimental value, fear of waste, or "what if I need it?" thinking.

- Acknowledge emotional attachments: It's okay to feel sentimental, but objects don't define memories; the experiences do.
- Reframe your mindset: Instead of thinking "I'm losing something", shift to "I'm making space for what truly matters."
- Give items a second life: Donate or repurpose them, knowing they will be used by someone who needs them.

Conclusion

Decluttering is a powerful tool for reducing stress, anxiety, and mental overload. Studies confirm that cleaner spaces improve mood, sleep quality, and productivity. By setting small goals, creating routines, and embracing a minimalist mindset, you can transform your home into a peaceful, organized space that supports mental well-being. Letting go of clutter isn't just about tidying; it's about making room for clarity, calmness, and a healthier mind.

12. Simplify Your Life

Overcommitment: Simplify Life and Reclaim Your Time

For years, I struggled with overcommitment: saying yes to too many responsibilities, trying to meet everyone's expectations, and filling my schedule to the point of exhaustion. I convinced myself that being busy meant being productive. But instead of feeling fulfilled, I felt stressed, drained, and disconnected from my own needs.

Overcommitment is a modern epidemic. Many people believe that doing more equals achieving more, but research suggests the opposite. Studies show that overcommitting leads to burnout, increased anxiety, reduced productivity, and lower overall life satisfaction (Leiter et al., 2014). In contrast, simplifying life and setting clear boundaries enhances mental health, work performance, and overall well-being (Schultz & Ryan, 2019).

This chapter explores how overcommitment affects mental health, why people feel compelled to take on too much, and provides practical strategies to simplify life and reclaim balance.

The Mental and Physical Toll of Overcommitment

Overcommitting is not just about having a busy schedule; it affects mental clarity, emotional well-being, and physical health.

1. Increased Stress and Anxiety
   - Research shows that people who overcommit experience significantly higher stress levels than those with structured, manageable schedules (Schultz & Ryan, 2019).
   - Chronically busy individuals have higher cortisol levels, leading to increased anxiety, irritability, and difficulty focusing (Leiter et al., 2014).
2. Burnout and Exhaustion
   - Taking on too many responsibilities can lead to physical and mental burnout. A study found that people who overcommit at work or in social life experience higher levels of exhaustion, reduced motivation, and emotional detachment (Maslach & Leiter, 2016).
   - Chronic burnout is associated with fatigue, insomnia, weakened immune function, and even heart disease (Bianchi et al., 2015).

3. Reduced Productivity and Decision Fatigue
   - People often think doing more means achieving more, but studies suggest that overloading your schedule decreases efficiency (Baumeister et al., 2007).
   - Decision fatigue, or mental exhaustion from making too many choices, reduces problem-solving skills, creativity, and overall productivity. (Vohs et al., 2014).
4. Neglecting Personal Well-Being
   - Overcommitment leads to neglect of self-care, sleep, and leisure, which are essential for long-term health and happiness.
   - Many overcommitted individuals struggle with poor eating habits, lack of exercise, and chronic fatigue, which contribute to mental and physical decline (Kabat-Zinn, 2013).

Why Do We Overcommit?

Understanding why we overcommit is the first step in breaking the cycle.

1. Fear of Saying No
   - Many people struggle with guilt or fear disappointing others when they decline commitments (Schultz & Ryan, 2019).
   - We believe that saying "no" makes us seem selfish, unhelpful, or unmotivated, even though it is necessary for mental balance.
2. The Illusion of Productivity
   - Society glorifies being busy, equating it with success. However, research shows that being constantly busy doesn't mean being effective (Newport, 2016).
   - Overcommitment leads to more distractions and unfinished projects, rather than meaningful accomplishments (Baumeister et al., 2007).
3. Social and Work Pressure
   - People feel pressure to please bosses, colleagues, family, and friends, making them say yes to commitments they don't truly have time for.
   - Workplace cultures that value "hustle" and overworking can make people feel guilty for setting limits, even when it negatively affects their health (Maslach & Leiter, 2016).
4, Avoidance of Personal Reflection

- Some people overcommit to avoid facing personal emotions, insecurities, or life challenges (Kabat-Zinn, 2013).
- Constant busyness provides a distraction from internal struggles, preventing meaningful self-growth.

How to Simplify Your Life and Reduce Overcommitment

1. Learn to Say No Without Guilt
   - Saying no is not selfish; it's self-care.
   - Use polite but firm responses:
     - *"I appreciate the offer, but I can't commit right now."*
     - *"I'd love to help, but my schedule is full at the moment."*
     - *"I need to prioritize my well-being, so I can't take this on right now."*
2. Prioritize What Truly Matters
   - Ask yourself:
     - *"Does this commitment align with my values and goals?"*
     - *"Is this something I truly want to do, or am I saying yes out of guilt?"*
     - *"Will this bring me joy or just add stress?"*
   - Focus on quality over quantity; commit to fewer things but give them your full energy.
3. Use the 80/20 Rule (Pareto Principle)
   - 80% of your happiness comes from 20% of your commitments; focus on what truly fulfills you (Koch, 2017).
   - Eliminate non-essential obligations that drain time and energy.
4. Schedule White Space in Your Calendar
   - Block out free time in your calendar for rest, hobbies, or relaxation, just as you would for meetings or work tasks. Avoid scheduling back-to-back activities; allow breathing room between tasks.
5. Stop multitasking; focus on one thing at a time
   - Studies show that multitasking reduces efficiency and increases stress (Levy et al., 2006).
   - Instead of juggling multiple commitments at once, focus on one task at a time.
6. Reduce Social Commitments That Drain You
   - If social gatherings or obligations feel forced or exhausting, limit them.
   - Surround yourself with people who energize you, not drain you.
7. Set Boundaries at Work and Home

- Avoid the trap of overworking to please others; set clear work-life boundaries.
- Communicate your limits: "I can't take on extra work at this time."
- Don't feel obligated to say yes to everything; your time is valuable.
- Simplify Your Daily Routines

8. Reduce decision fatigue by simplifying daily habits:
- Plan meals in advance.
- Choose a minimalist wardrobe to avoid outfit stress.
- Automate tasks (bill payments, grocery deliveries, etc.).

9. Embrace "JOMO" (Joy of Missing Out)
- Instead of fearing missing out (FOMO), embrace JOMO; the joy of doing less.
- Appreciate quiet moments, rest, and simplicity.

10. Reflect and Adjust Regularly

Every month, review your commitments and ask:
- *"What can I remove from my schedule?"*
- *"Am I prioritizing my health and happiness?"*
- *"Do I feel fulfilled or just exhausted?"*

Conclusion

Overcommitment leads to stress, burnout, and reduced quality of life. However, simplifying your schedule, setting boundaries, and focusing on what truly matters can help you reclaim your time and mental well-being. By learning to say no, prioritize meaningful commitments, and embrace a slower pace, you can create a balanced, fulfilling life that nurtures both productivity and peace.

13. Mindfulness and Meditation

13. Mindfulness and Meditation

The Power of a Few Minutes: Why Daily Meditation Matters

In the fast-paced, overstimulated world we live in, the idea of sitting still in silence may seem unproductive or even unnecessary. But research consistently shows that setting aside just a few minutes each day for meditation can have profound effects on mental health, emotional regulation, and even brain function. You don't need hours of silence; just a few intentional minutes can begin to shift your mental state, helping calm the nervous system, reduce stress hormones, and rewire patterns of negative thinking that fuel depression.

Numerous studies have confirmed the benefits of even short daily meditation practices. A randomized controlled trial published in *JAMA Internal Medicine* found that participants who engaged in mindfulness meditation for just 20 minutes a day experienced significant reductions in symptoms of anxiety and depression compared to a control group (Goyal et al., 2014). Another study using functional MRI scans showed that brief daily mindfulness sessions (as short as 13 minutes) led to reduced amygdala activation, the part of the brain responsible for stress and fear responses, and increased connectivity in areas involved in emotional regulation and self-awareness (Taren et al., 2015). These neurological changes mirror what many people report after consistent practice: greater calm, improved focus, and a stronger sense of control over their thoughts.

What makes meditation especially powerful for individuals with depression is its ability to break the cycle of rumination, the repetitive, negative thought loops that reinforce hopelessness and despair. Meditation helps create psychological distance between you and your thoughts, allowing you to observe them without getting pulled into their narrative. Over time, this process, known as cognitive defusion, reduces the emotional grip of negative thinking and fosters a more grounded, balanced internal state.

Even five minutes a day can serve as a reset for the brain. It's not about achieving perfect stillness or emptying the mind, but about building the habit of tuning in and cultivating awareness. Just as physical exercise strengthens the body, meditation strengthens the mind's resilience and flexibility. Making time for daily meditation, no matter how short, is a powerful investment in your long-term emotional well-being and an essential tool in your recovery journey.

Mindfulness and Simple Breathing Meditation: Finding Peace in the Present

For years, I lived in a constant state of stress, overthinking, and mental exhaustion. My mind was always racing: worrying about the future, replaying past mistakes, or planning my next task. I thought I needed to do more, think more, and push harder to stay in control. But the truth was, I was never fully present, and it was draining me.

Then, I discovered mindfulness, the practice of being fully aware of the present moment without judgment. It helped me quiet my mind, reduce anxiety, and find clarity in ways I never thought possible. Studies show that mindfulness and meditation reduce stress, enhance emotional regulation, and improve overall well-being (Kabat-Zinn, 2013).

What Is Mindfulness?

Mindfulness is the practice of paying full attention to the present moment without trying to change it. It means observing your thoughts, emotions, and sensations without reacting to them (Brown & Ryan, 2003). Instead of dwelling on the past or worrying about the future, mindfulness trains the brain to stay present, accepting things as they are.

How Mindfulness Benefits Mental Health

1. Reduces Stress and Anxiety: Mindfulness lowers cortisol levels, the hormone linked to stress and anxiety (Tang et al., 2015). Studies show that meditation-based mindfulness training significantly reduces chronic stress and improves mental resilience (Goyal et al., 2014).
2. Improves Emotional Regulation: Practicing mindfulness reduces emotional reactivity, allowing you to respond to situations calmly rather than impulsively (Hölzel et al., 2011). It strengthens self-awareness, helping you recognize and process emotions more effectively.
3. Enhances Focus and Cognitive Function: Mindfulness increases gray matter density in brain regions associated with attention and decision-making (Tang et al., 2015).

Regular practice improves memory, concentration, and problem-solving skills (Zeidan et al., 2010).
4. Promotes Better Sleep: Mindfulness calms the nervous system, making it easier to fall asleep and stay asleep (Ong et al., 2014). Meditation before bed reduces racing thoughts and nighttime anxiety.

Simple Breathing Meditation for Calm and Clarity

One of the easiest and most effective mindfulness practices is breathing meditation. By focusing on your breath, you train your mind to stay present and let go of distractions.

1. Basic Breathing Meditation (5 Minutes)

Step 1: Find a quiet, comfortable space to sit. Keep your spine straight but relaxed.
Step 2: Close your eyes and bring your attention to your breath.
Step 3: Breathe in slowly through your nose, feeling your belly expand.
Step 4: Exhale gently through your mouth, feeling tension leave your body.
Step 5: If your mind wanders, gently bring it back to the breath.
   Tip: Set a timer for 5 minutes and gradually increase to 10–15 minutes over time.

2. The 4-7-8 Relaxation Breath (For Stress Relief)

A powerful technique for calming the nervous system.
Step 1: Inhale deeply through your nose for 4 seconds.
Step 2: Hold your breath for 7 seconds.
Step 3: Slowly exhale through your mouth for 8 seconds.
Step 4: Repeat for 4 rounds.
   Best for: Reducing stress, improving sleep, calming anxiety.

3. Box Breathing (For Focus and Clarity)

A technique used by Navy SEALs to enhance concentration under pressure.
Step 1: Inhale for 4 seconds.
Step 2: Hold the breath for 4 seconds.

Step 3: Exhale for 4 seconds.
Step 4: Hold again for 4 seconds.
Step 5: Repeat for 5 minutes.

✅ Best for: Enhancing focus, relieving anxiety, preparing for high-stress situations.

4. Mindful Walking (For Mental Clarity)

Instead of walking on autopilot, turn it into a grounding mindfulness practice.
Step 1: Walk slowly and intentionally, feeling the movement of your feet.
Step 2: Focus on the sensation of your breath, the wind, and the ground beneath you.
Step 3: Observe your surroundings without judgment.
Step 4: If your mind wanders, gently bring it back to the present.

✅ Best for: Reducing stress, clearing the mind, breaking up long work sessions.

5. Body Scan Meditation (For Deep Relaxation)

Helps release physical tension and stress stored in the body.
Step 1: Lie down in a comfortable position.
Step 2: Close your eyes and take a deep breath.
Step 3: Slowly bring your attention to each body part, starting from your feet and moving upwards.
Step 4: Notice any tension or discomfort, and consciously relax that area.
Step 5: Finish by taking three deep breaths and slowly opening your eyes.

✅ Best for: Relaxation, reducing muscle tension, preparing for sleep.

How to Make Mindfulness a Daily Habit

◆ Start small: Just 5 minutes a day can make a difference.

◆ Pair it with daily routines: Meditate after waking up or before bedtime.

◆ Use reminders: Set phone alerts or place sticky notes as mindfulness cues.

◆ Be patient: Mindfulness is a skill that improves with practice.

Conclusion

Mindfulness is a simple yet powerful tool that helps you reduce stress, improve focus, and find peace in the present moment. Through breathing exercises, meditation, and mindful movement, you can cultivate a calm, centered mind. By practicing mindfulness daily, you can train your brain to be less reactive, more present, and more resilient, creating a life of greater clarity, peace, and emotional balance.

14. Behavior Modification

Behavior Modification: The Key to Lasting Change

After years of struggling with stress, overcommitment, screen addiction, clutter, and unhealthy habits, I realized that willpower alone wasn't enough to make lasting changes. No matter how determined I was, I often fell back into old patterns. The real key to transformation wasn't just knowing what to do; it was learning how to change behavior effectively.

Behavior modification is the science of changing habits by understanding triggers, reinforcing positive actions, and creating sustainable routines (Skinner, 1953). Research shows that small, intentional behavior shifts, rather than extreme, unsustainable efforts, lead to lasting improvements in mental health, productivity, and well-being (Wood & Neal, 2007).

This chapter wraps up everything we've discussed, including overcoming stress, reducing overcommitment, limiting screen time, decluttering, and simplifying life, by focusing on practical strategies for long-term behavior change.

Why Behavior Modification Works

Breaking bad habits and building better ones isn't just about motivation; it's about understanding how habits work and changing them at their source.

Habits Are Automatic

Studies show that 40–50% of our daily actions are habitual, meaning they happen without conscious thought (Neal et al., 2006). Changing habits requires rewiring the brain by modifying triggers and rewards.

Willpower Alone Is Not Enough

Research shows that willpower is a limited resource; it depletes over time (Baumeister et al., 1998). Instead of relying on sheer effort, behavior modification uses systems and routines to make habits easier to sustain.

Consistency Beats Intensity

Small, consistent changes over time are more effective than extreme efforts that fizzle out (Lally et al., 2010). Example: Five minutes of decluttering daily is more sustainable than trying to clean the entire house in one exhausting session.

Practical Behavior Modification Strategies

1. Identify Your Triggers and Replace the Routine
Example: Screen Time
> Trigger: Feeling bored → Routine: Mindlessly scrolling social media
> Modification: When feeling bored, replace scrolling with reading a book or stretching

Example: Overcommitment
> Trigger: Fear of disappointing others → Routine: Saying yes to everything
> Modification: Pause and ask *"Do I really want this?"* before responding

2. Start Small (The 2-Minute Rule)
> Research shows that habits are easier to stick to when they start small (Fogg, 2020).
> Example: Instead of committing to 30 minutes of meditation daily, start with 2-4 minutes. Once the habit is established, build on it.

3. Use Habit Stacking
> Attach a new habit to an existing one to make it easier to follow (Clear, 2018).
> Example:
> *"After I brush my teeth, I will do 2 minutes of deep breathing."*
> *"After I make my morning coffee, I will write down 3 things I'm grateful for."*

4. Make It Easy and Remove Friction
Example: Reducing Screen Time
> Hard Version: "I will stop using my phone so much."
> Easier Version: "I will delete social media apps from my home screen to reduce temptation."

Example: Decluttering
> Hard Version: "I will clean my entire house this weekend."
> Easier Version: "I will remove one item I don't need every day."

5. Set Clear Boundaries and Say No
> People who set clear personal and work boundaries experience lower stress and better life balance (Schultz & Ryan, 2019).

Examples:
> Limit social events to two per week.
> Set a "no email after 7 PM" rule to improve work-life balance.

6. Use Rewards to Reinforce Good Behavior

Our brains respond to positive reinforcement (Skinner, 1953).
Examples:

> Reward yourself with a favorite podcast episode after completing a difficult task. Give yourself a day off social media after a week of consistent exercise or decluttering.

7. Track Progress and Celebrate Small Wins

> Studies show that habit tracking increases success rates (Lally et al., 2010). Use a journal, calendar, or app to monitor progress.

Example:

> Check off days with limited screen time or when you've said no to unnecessary commitments.

8. Create a Supportive Environment

> Surround yourself with people who support your goals (Christakis & Fowler, 2007).

Example:

> If you want to declutter, join a minimalist group for motivation.
> If you're reducing screen time, have a friend hold you accountable.

9. Practice Self-Compassion

> Studies show that self-criticism weakens motivation, while self-compassion improves resilience (Neff, 2011). If you miss a day or fall back into old habits, don't quit; just restart.

Here are practical behavior modification strategies for each of the 14 secrets for anxiety and depression, designed to be actionable and simple enough to implement daily. These suggestions align with behavior change science and are geared toward long-term mental wellness.

1. Food and Depression

Behavior Strategy: Start with one anti-inflammatory meal per day. For example, swap processed snacks for a bowl of berries and nuts. Build consistency before making broader dietary changes. Check *Eat to Heal* for more details on a detailed anti-inflammatory diet.

2. Vitamins, Minerals, and Hormone Imbalance

Behavior Strategy: Consult a clinical nutritionist practitioner to evaluate potential deficiencies and receive personalized dosage recommendations. Once assessed, set a daily reminder to take your supplements and use a pill organizer to stay consistent. Pair supplement intake with an existing habit, such as brushing your teeth or eating breakfast.

3. Drug-Induced Depression
Behavior Strategy: Track mood changes in a journal or app after starting any new medication. Share patterns with your healthcare provider. Always review side effects and alternatives with your doctor.

4. Brain Glitches: Your Thoughts Are Not You
Behavior Strategy: Use the "name the thought" technique. When a negative thought appears, label it ("There's the critic") and let it pass instead of engaging. Practice for 2 minutes daily.

5. Distance Yourself & Zoom Out
Behavior Strategy: Schedule a weekly 10-minute "mental zoom-out" session. Write down a problem and ask yourself: "How will I see this in 1 year?" or "What advice would I give a friend in this situation?"

6. Trauma Closure: BioPsycho Therapy (BPT)
Behavior Strategy: It is important to address proper trauma closure through internal healing techniques such as BioPsycho Therapy, which integrates both the psychological and physiological aspects of trauma for lasting recovery.

7. The Illusion of Control
Behavior Strategy: List 3 things outside your control and 3 within it each morning. Focus your action only on what's in your control. This reinforces acceptance and directs energy productively.

8. Change Is the Only Constant
Behavior Strategy: Reflect weekly on one recent change and write what you learned from it. This builds resilience and rewires your brain to associate change with growth.

9. Forgiveness

Behavior Strategy: Write a 5-minute letter of forgiveness (you don't have to send it). Do this once a week. This helps to release emotional tension and builds empathy over time.

10. Limit Screen Time
Behavior Strategy: Set a screen curfew 1 hour before bed. Replace that time with a calming routine like stretching, reading, or reflection. Use screen timers or grayscale mode on your phone to support the habit.

11. Declutter Your Home
Behavior Strategy: Start with 5 minutes a day. Choose one drawer, shelf, or surface. Set a timer, remove items, and ask, "Do I use or love this?" Make it part of your morning or evening wind-down.

12. Simplify Your Life
Behavior Strategy: Every Sunday, write down 3 commitments you can cancel, delegate, or say no to. This weekly reset builds space and reduces overwhelm.

13. Mindfulness and Meditation
Behavior Strategy: Start with 2 minutes of mindful breathing after waking up. Use a timer or an app with gentle sounds. Gradually increase as it becomes a habit.

14. Behavior Modification
Behavior Strategy: Use the "cue–routine–reward" model. Identify a habit you want to build (e.g., going for a walk), pair it with an existing routine (e.g., after lunch), and follow it with a reward (e.g., tea or music). Track your progress daily.

Even God, in His infinite power, created the earth in six days and intentionally set aside the seventh day for rest, signifying the essential balance between work and rejuvenation. This divine pattern serves as a profound reminder that sustained productivity and creativity depend not only on continuous effort but also on purposeful rest. In my own experience, I am often consumed by a relentless cycle of inventing new medical devices, meticulously researching scientific studies, or deeply engrossed in writing my next book. These passions frequently lead me to overlook the necessity of a dedicated day off, ultimately risking burnout and diminishing the quality of my endeavors.

Recognizing the significance of rest as demonstrated in the act of creation itself, I have committed to intentionally setting aside one day each week solely for relaxation and reflection. On this day, I consciously limit my phone usage and significantly reduce screen time, allowing my mind to disconnect fully from the demands and distractions of technology. Instead, I devote this sacred time to meditation, enjoying rejuvenating moments in nature, and creating meaningful memories with my family. This intentional practice of slowing down, reflecting, and reconnecting provides an opportunity to recharge mentally, emotionally, and physically. By following this purposeful rhythm, directly inspired by the Creator Himself, I honor my health, enrich my relationships, enhance my productivity, and cultivate greater balance and harmony in my personal and professional life.

Conclusion

For years, I struggled with depression, anxiety, PTSD and overwhelming stress. I searched for solutions, only to find that traditional treatments often focused on symptoms rather than root causes. Through my personal journey and my work with patients, I discovered that true healing is multifaceted; it requires addressing not just the mind, but the body and lifestyle as well. This book has explored 14 powerful secrets that have helped me and many others overcome depression and reclaim our well-being. Each chapter has provided scientific insights, practical strategies, and proven methods to help you transform your mental health naturally. Let's take a final look at these 14 key secrets and how they work together as a comprehensive healing approach.

1. Inflammatory Food: Healing Through Nutrition

What we eat directly impacts our brain function, mood, and overall mental health. Chronic inflammation from processed foods, sugar, and toxins can contribute to depression and anxiety. The ASTR Diet, which I developed, focuses on anti-inflammatory, sustainable, toxin-free, and restorative foods to nourish both body and mind. Check *Eat to Heal* for more details on a detailed anti-inflammatory diet.

◆ Takeaway: Eliminate inflammatory foods and adopt a healing, whole-food diet for long-term mental and physical well-being.

2. Drug-Induced Depression: Understanding Hidden Triggers

Many people don't realize that common medications, including those for blood pressure, birth control, and even pain relief, can disrupt neurotransmitter balance and contribute to depression. Understanding the side effects of medications and working with a qualified healthcare provider can prevent unnecessary suffering.

◆ Takeaway: Always review medications with a healthcare professional and consider natural alternatives when possible.

3. Vitamins, Minerals, and Hormone Imbalances: The Missing Link

Depression is often mistakenly linked solely to neurotransmitter imbalances, but the truth is that the brain can't produce neurotransmitters without essential nutrients. Deficiencies in iron, magnesium, zinc, and B vitamins can lead to fatigue, low mood, and brain fog. Through both my personal experience and my clinical practice, I've seen that most patients with depression have at least 4 to 8 nutrient deficiencies. Consult a clinical nutritionist practitioner to evaluate potential deficiencies and receive personalized dosage recommendations. Once assessed, set a daily reminder to take your supplements and use a pill organizer to stay consistent. Pair supplement intake with an existing habit, such as brushing your teeth or eating breakfast.

◆ Takeaway: Work with a clinical nutritionist to identify and correct nutrient imbalances; your brain needs the right building blocks to function optimally.

4. Brain Glitches: Your Thoughts Are Not You
Our brains constantly generate thoughts, but not all of them are real or meaningful. Intrusive, irrational, or negative thoughts are not a reflection of reality; they are simply brain glitches that can be observed and dismissed. Understanding this helps reduce fear and emotional distress.

◆ Takeaway: Train yourself to recognize irrational thoughts and detach from them instead of believing or engaging with them.

5. Distance Yourself: Zoom Out from Negative Thoughts
Negative thoughts can feel overwhelming, but they only have power if we engage with them. A key strategy is to mentally step back, observe thoughts like scenes in a movie, and avoid fueling them with attention.

◆ Takeaway: Instead of getting lost in thoughts, watch them from a distance and let them pass without reaction.

6. The Illusion of Control: Letting Go for Inner Peace
Many of us live under the illusion that we can control everything: our environment, other people, and even random events. This leads to stress, frustration, and anxiety. In reality, the only thing we can control is our own actions and mindset.

◆ Takeaway: Focus on what you can control (your responses, actions, and mindset) and let go of external factors beyond your influence.

7. Trauma Closure: BPT (Biopsycho Therapy)
It is important to address proper trauma closure through internal healing techniques such as BioPsycho Therapy, which integrates both the psychological and physiological aspects of trauma for lasting recovery.

◆ Takeaway: Healing from trauma requires closure. The only realistic closure we can achieve is internal, and using the BPT approach is a powerful way to get there.

8. Change Is the Only Constant
Resisting change often leads to anxiety, frustration, and a sense of helplessness. Yet, change is a natural and unavoidable part of life. Learning to accept and adapt to change fosters resilience, flexibility, and personal growth.

◆ Takeaway: Reframe change as an opportunity for growth rather than a threat. Build resilience by reflecting on how you've grown through past transitions.

9. Forgiveness
Holding onto resentment, anger, or guilt can create chronic emotional stress, which negatively affects mental and physical health. Forgiveness isn't about excusing harmful behavior; it's about releasing the burden and reclaiming peace of mind. Letting go frees up emotional energy and promotes healing.

◆ Takeaway: Practice forgiveness regularly, whether through journaling, reflection, or therapy. Releasing past pain creates space for emotional freedom and growth.

10. Limiting Screen Time
Excessive screen time, especially on social media, has been linked to depression, anxiety, and poor sleep. Constant digital stimulation overstimulates the brain, disrupting focus, emotional balance, and sleep quality.

◆ Takeaway: Reduce screen time, set boundaries on social media use, and prioritize real-world connections for better mental health.

11. Declutter Your House: Clearing Mental and Physical Space
Cluttered environments contribute to stress, anxiety, and decision fatigue. Studies show that clean, organized spaces improve mood, sleep quality, and cognitive function.

◆ Takeaway: Declutter one space at a time, simplifying your home to reduce stress and create a calming environment.

12. Overcommitment: Simplify Life for Mental Clarity

Saying yes to everything leads to stress, burnout, and loss of personal time. Society glorifies busyness, but true well-being comes from setting boundaries and prioritizing what truly matters.

◆ Takeaway: Learn to say no without guilt and simplify your schedule for a more peaceful, fulfilling life.

13. Meditation & Mindfulness:
Breathing techniques and mindfulness activate the parasympathetic nervous system, reducing stress, anxiety, and intrusive thoughts. Practicing deep breathing, box breathing, and body scan meditation can instantly shift your mental state from chaos to calm.

◆ Takeaway: Use simple breathing exercises and mindfulness practices daily to create a sense of peace and presence.

14. Behavior Modification: The Key to Lasting Change
Knowing what to do is not enough; you need systems to make healthy habits automatic. Using habit stacking, small daily actions, and positive reinforcement helps create sustainable mental and physical health improvements.

◆ Takeaway: Focus on small, consistent changes, and use behavior modification strategies to make new habits stick for life.

Your Path Forward: Putting It All Together

Healing is a journey, not a quick fix. Each of these 14 secrets contributes to restoring balance to your mind and body. By applying one step at a time, you will begin to see real improvements in your mental health, energy levels, and overall well-being.

Remember:

✅ **Start small:** Choose one or two changes to implement today.

✅ **Be patient:** Lasting transformation takes time.

✅ **Listen to your body and mind:** Your needs may change over time.

✅ **Seek support:** Whether through a community, therapist, or healthcare provider.

Conclusion

I know from experience that healing is possible. By addressing inflammation, vitamin and mineral deficiencies, understanding brain glitches, distancing yourself from negative thoughts, practicing meditation, cultivating a healthy mindset, improving lifestyle habits, and setting personal boundaries, you can break free from depression and anxiety and step into a life of clarity, peace, and vitality. Your journey starts now; take the first step today.

You deserve a life free from depression, chronic stress, and emotional turmoil. By following the principles in this book, you are giving yourself the gift of healing, empowerment, and resilience. Thank you for taking this journey with me. I hope these tools help you transform your life as they did mine.

Recommended Resources

How to Access Online Content
1. Open the camera app on your smartphone.
2. Point the camera at the barcode.
3. A notification will appear with a link. Tap the notification to open the link in your browser.

1. Case Studies

2. <u>Limited Time Offer</u>: FREE 30-minute Health Coach Consultation

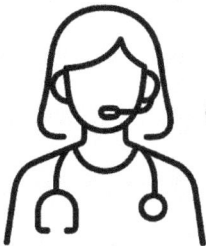

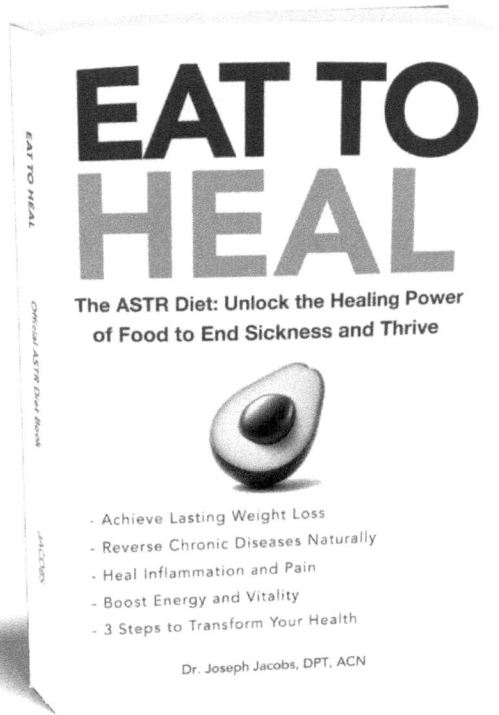

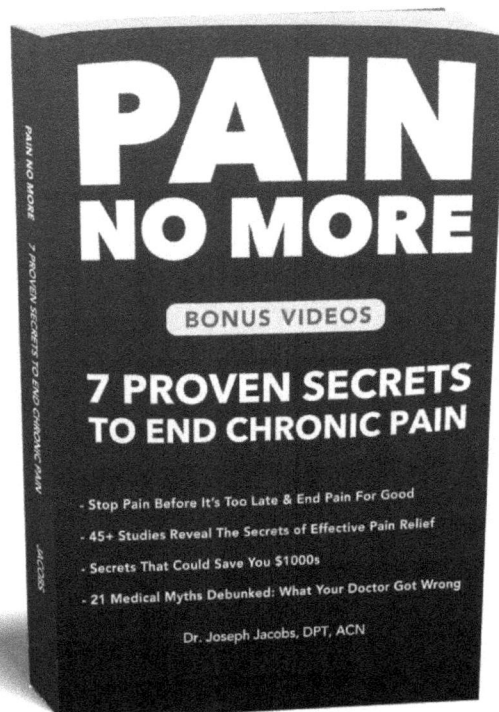

BEATING
MIGRAINES

BONUS VIDEOS

7 NATURAL SECRETS FOR
LASTING RELIEF

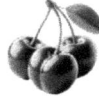

- End Migraines Naturally
- Clinically Proven Methods
- Treat the Root Cause, Not Symptoms
- Insights from a Doctor & Migraine Survivor
- Research-Backed Relief for Life

Dr. Joseph Jacobs, DPT, ACN

BEATING
BACK PAIN

BONUS VIDEOS

7 NATURAL SECRETS FOR
LASTING RELIEF

- End Back Pain Naturally
- Clinically Tested, Doctor-Approved
- Fix the Root Causes, Not Just Symptoms
- Backed by Science & Research
- Created by a Doctor Who Beat Chronic Pain

Dr. Joseph Jacobs, DPT, ACN

REVERSING
HIGH BLOOD
PRESSURE

7 NATURAL SECRETS TO SAFELY
LOWER BLOOD PRESSURE

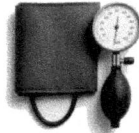

- Natural Solutions That Work
- Backed by Extensive Research
- Fix the Root Cause, Not Just the Numbers
- No Drugs, No Side Effects

Dr. Joseph Jacobs, DPT, ACN

REVERSING
DIABETES

10 NATURAL SECRETS TO REVERSE
DIABETES WITHOUT DRUGS

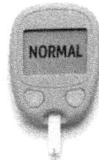

NORMAL

- Drug-Free, Side-Effect-Free, Science-Backed Healing
- Treat the Root Cause, Not Just the Symptoms
- Proven Natural Strategies That Get Results

Dr. Joseph Jacobs, DPT, ACN

KILLED BY FRAGRANCE

How Synthetic Scents Make Us Sick

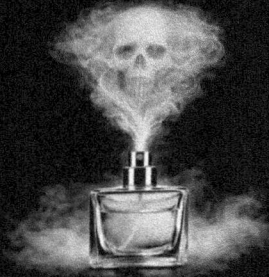

- Exposed by peer-reviewed research
- Links everyday fragrance exposure to chronic disease
- Built on science, not opinion

Dr. Joseph Jacobs, DPT, ACN

Your SHOES HURT YOU

Why Does Your Pain Keep Coming Back and *How to Fix It*

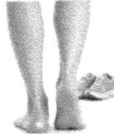

BONUS VIDEOS

- Fix Your Feet. Fix Your Pain.
- Why Modern Shoes Create Chronic Pain
- Backed by Biomechanics and Clinical Research

Dr. Joseph Jacobs, DPT, ACN

Glossary

Agoraphobia
An anxiety disorder characterized by the fear of being in situations where escape might be difficult or help unavailable. Individuals often avoid crowded places, open spaces, or situations where they feel trapped.

Amygdala
A key brain structure involved in processing emotions, particularly fear and threat detection. Overactivity of the amygdala is linked to anxiety, PTSD, and emotional dysregulation.

Anxiety
A physiological and emotional response to perceived threats. While normal in small amounts, chronic anxiety leads to excessive worry, nervousness, and physical symptoms such as rapid heart rate and tension.

Anti-Inflammatory Diet
A nutritional approach emphasizing foods that reduce systemic inflammation, including fruits, vegetables, healthy fats, and lean proteins, while avoiding processed foods, refined sugars, and trans fats.

ASTR Diet
A balanced, anti-inflammatory, toxin-free, sustainable, and restorative dietary protocol developed to promote healing, reduce chronic inflammation, and support emotional well-being.

BioPsycho Therapy (BPT)
A trauma-informed treatment approach combining magnetic stimulation and exposure therapy techniques to release stored trauma from the nervous system, facilitating trauma closure and emotional recovery.

Brain Glitches
Distorted or exaggerated thought patterns that misrepresent reality, contributing to anxiety and depression. Recognizing brain glitches helps individuals distance themselves from negative thought loops.

Cognitive Defusion
A psychological skill that teaches individuals to detach from their thoughts, recognizing them as temporary mental events rather than absolute truths.

Cortisol
A hormone released during the body's stress response. Chronic high cortisol levels can damage brain structures involved in mood regulation and lead to anxiety, depression, and fatigue.

Decluttering
The act of organizing and removing unnecessary possessions from one's living environment to reduce mental stress, improve focus, and promote emotional clarity.

Depression
A symptom (not a disease) characterized by persistent sadness, loss of interest, fatigue, and impaired cognitive and emotional function. Depression often arises from underlying physiological dysfunctions.

Fight-or-Flight Response
The body's automatic survival response triggered by perceived threats, preparing the individual to fight or flee. Chronic activation of this response contributes to anxiety disorders and health issues.

Forgiveness
The process of releasing resentment, anger, and blame toward oneself or others. Forgiveness is essential for emotional healing and is linked to reduced depression and stress levels.

Glossary

Generalized Anxiety Disorder (GAD)
A type of anxiety disorder involving persistent and excessive worry about everyday life situations, lasting for at least six months and significantly impairing daily functioning.

Gut-Brain Axis
The communication system between the gastrointestinal tract and the brain. Disruptions in gut health, such as imbalanced gut microbiota, can contribute to inflammation and mental health disorders.

HPA Axis (Hypothalamic-Pituitary-Adrenal Axis)
A major neuroendocrine system involved in the body's response to stress. Dysregulation of the HPA axis can lead to mood disorders, chronic fatigue, and weakened immune function.

Hypothyroidism
A condition in which the thyroid gland does not produce enough hormones, leading to symptoms like fatigue, weight gain, and depression.

Inflammation
The body's natural defense response to injury or infection. Chronic, low-grade inflammation is linked to depression, anxiety, and other chronic diseases.

Magnesium Deficiency
A lack of adequate magnesium, a mineral vital for stress regulation, neurotransmitter function, and nervous system health. Magnesium deficiency is linked to anxiety, depression, and sleep disorders.

Mindfulness
A practice of nonjudgmental awareness of the present moment, fostering emotional regulation, reduced anxiety, and improved resilience.

Neurotransmitters
Chemical messengers in the brain, such as serotonin, dopamine, and norepinephrine, that regulate mood, energy, motivation, and emotional stability.

Nutritional Psychiatry
A field of research and clinical practice that focuses on the impact of diet and nutrition on mental health outcomes, emphasizing nutrient-rich, anti-inflammatory foods.

Panic Attack
A sudden, intense episode of fear or discomfort, often accompanied by physical symptoms like chest pain, dizziness, heart palpitations, and shortness of breath.

Persistent Depressive Disorder (PDD)
Also known as dysthymia, a chronic form of depression lasting for at least two years, characterized by persistent low mood and feelings of hopelessness.

Post-Traumatic Stress Disorder (PTSD)
A psychiatric condition triggered by experiencing or witnessing traumatic events. Symptoms include flashbacks, emotional numbness, hypervigilance, and avoidance behaviors.

Prefrontal Cortex
The part of the brain responsible for executive functions such as planning, decision-making, emotional regulation, and social behavior. Dysfunction in this area is associated with depression and anxiety.

Processed Foods
Foods altered through manufacturing processes that often contain high levels of sugar, trans fats, preservatives, and additives, all of which contribute to inflammation and worsen mental health.

Screen Time
Time spent using devices with screens such as smartphones, computers, and televisions. Excessive screen time has been linked to increased rates of anxiety, depression, and sleep disturbances.

Glossary

Serotonin
A neurotransmitter involved in mood regulation, sleep, and appetite. Low serotonin levels have traditionally been associated with depression, although newer research suggests nutrient deficiencies play a larger role.

Simplification
The process of streamlining life activities, obligations, and possessions to reduce stress, enhance focus, and improve emotional well-being.

Specific Phobia
An intense, irrational fear of a specific object, situation, or activity that poses little or no actual danger.

Stress Response System
The biological system involving the brain and body's reactions to perceived stress, primarily mediated through the HPA axis, cortisol release, and sympathetic nervous system activation.

Sympathetic Nervous System
The branch of the autonomic nervous system responsible for activating the "fight-or-flight" response during perceived threats.

Trauma Closure
The resolution of unprocessed traumatic memories and emotional wounds stored in the nervous system, critical for long-term recovery from PTSD, anxiety, and depression.

Vitamin D Deficiency
Low levels of vitamin D, a hormone essential for brain health, immune regulation, and mood stability. Deficiency is associated with depression, fatigue, and weakened immunity.

Vitamin and Mineral Deficiencies
Insufficient levels of essential nutrients critical for neurotransmitter synthesis, brain health, and emotional stability. Common deficiencies include magnesium, B vitamins, vitamin D, and omega-3 fatty acids.

References

1. Feldman R, Eidelman AI. The neurobiology of depression. Nat Rev Neurosci. 2020;21(2):63-80.
2. Krishnan V, Nestler EJ. The molecular neurobiology of depression. Nature. 2018;455(7215):894-902.
3. Moret C, Briley M. The importance of norepinephrine in depression. Neuropsychiatr Dis Treat. 2019;15:2055-2065.
4. Pariante CM. Why are depressed patients inflamed? A neuroimmune perspective. Trends Immunol. 2017;38(1):46-57.
5. Yehuda R, Hoge CW, McFarlane AC, Vermetten E, Lanius RA. Post-traumatic stress disorder. Nat Rev Dis Primers.2015;1:15057.
6. World Health Organization. Depression. Published 2023. Accessed March 10, 2024. https://www.who.int/news-room/fact-sheets/detail/depression
7. National Institute of Mental Health. Major Depression. Published 2022. Accessed March 10, 2024. https://www.nimh.nih.gov/health/statistics/major-depression
8. Anxiety and Depression Association of America. Facts and Statistics. Published 2022. Accessed March 10, 2024. https://adaa.org/finding-help/helpful-resources/facts-statistics
9. Chisholm D, Sweeny K, Sheehan P, et al. Scaling-up treatment of depression and anxiety: A global return on investment analysis. Lancet Psychiatry. 2016;3(5):415-424.
10. Stewart WF, Ricci JA, Chee E, Hahn SR, Morganstein D. Cost of lost productive work time among US workers with depression. JAMA. 2003;289(23):3135-3144.
11. Akbaraly TN, Sabia S, Hagger-Johnson G, et al. Does overall diet in midlife predict future depressive symptoms? Br J Psychiatry. 2018;203(5):357-364.
12. Cattaneo A, Ferrari C, Turner L, et al. Whole-blood expression of inflammation-related genes in depression and the response to antidepressants. Transl Psychiatry. 2020;10(1):3.
13. Jacka FN, O'Neil A, Opie R, et al. A randomised controlled trial of dietary improvement for adults with major depression (the 'SMILES' trial). BMC Med. 2017;15(1):23.
14. Knüppel A, Shipley MJ, Llewellyn CH, Brunner EJ. Sugar intake from sweet food and beverages, common mental disorder and depression. Sci Rep. 2017;7:6287.
15. Sánchez-Villegas A, Zazpe I, Santiago S, et al. Energy and nutrient intake and risk of depression in the SUN project. BMC Psychiatry. 2019;13(1):1-9.
16. Anglin RE, Samaan Z, Walter SD, McDonald SD. Vitamin D deficiency and depression in adults. J Affect Disord.2013;150(2):268-278.
17. Boyle NB, Lawton C, Dye L. The effects of magnesium supplementation on subjective anxiety and stress. Nutrients.2017;9(5):429.
18. Tarleton EK, Littenberg B, MacLean CD, Kennedy AG, Daley C. Magnesium intake and depression in adults. J Am Board Fam Med. 2017;30(4):521-530.
19. Kaplan BJ, Rucklidge JJ, Romijn AR, McLeod K. The emerging field of nutritional mental health. Clin Psychol Sci.2015;3(6):964-980.
20. Penninx BW, Guralnik JM, Ferrucci L, Fried LP, Allen RH, Stabler SP. Vitamin B12 deficiency and depression. Arch Gen Psychiatry. 2016;57(1):85-92.
21. Wilkins CH, Sheline YI, Roe CM, Birge SJ, Morris JC. Vitamin D deficiency associated with depression in older adults. Am J Geriatr Psychiatry. 2016;14(12):1032-1040.
22. Nowak G, Szewczyk B, Pilc A. Zinc and depression. Pharmacol Rep. 2018;65(3):545-558.
23. Tarleton EK, Littenberg B. Magnesium intake and depression in adults. J Am Board Fam Med. 2017;30(4):521-530.

References

24. Swardfager W, Herrmann N, McIntyre RS, et al. Zinc in depression: a meta-analysis. Biol Psychiatry.2013;74(12):872-878.
25. Zhao L, Bao H, Peng S, et al. Association of iron deficiency anemia with depressive symptoms in Chinese women. Psychiatry Res. 2018;267:631-636.
26. Spinneker A, Sola R, Lemmen V, Castillo MJ, Pietrzik K, Gonzalez-Gross M. Vitamin B6 status, deficiency and its consequences—an overview. Nutr Hosp. 2007;22(1):7-24.
27. Schwalfenberg GK, Genuis SJ. The importance of magnesium in clinical healthcare. Scientifica (Cairo).2017;2017:4179326. doi:10.1155/2017/4179326.
28. Kharbanda KK. Iron imbalance and alcohol-induced liver damage: role of hepcidin. Biomolecules. 2022;12(1):1-12. doi:10.3390/biom12010001.
29. Bertinato J, Zouzoulas A, Lavergne C, et al. Excess zinc supplementation disrupts zinc homeostasis, impairs bone health and affects the gut microbiota in rats. Nutrients. 2021;13(4):1261. doi:10.3390/nu13041261.
30. National Institutes of Health. Office of Dietary Supplements: Magnesium. Updated March 29, 2023. Accessed March 12, 2024. https://ods.od.nih.gov/factsheets/Magnesium-HealthProfessional/
31. Fava M, Rush AJ, Thase ME. Treatment-resistant depression: impact of medications on neurobiological mechanisms. Mol Psychiatry. 2018;23(2):234-243.
32. Skovlund CW, Morch LS, Kessing LV, Lidegaard O. Association of hormonal contraception with depression. JAMA Psychiatry. 2016;73(11):1154-1162.
33. Scherrer JF, Salas J, Copeland LA, Stock EM, Schneider FD. Prescription opioid duration, dose, and depression. Ann Fam Med. 2016;14(1):54-62.
34. Brewin CR, Gregory JD, Lipton M, Burgess N. Intrusive memories in PTSD. Nat Rev Neurosci. 2010;11(3):181-190.
35. LeDoux J. Anxious: Using the Brain to Understand and Treat Fear and Anxiety. Penguin Random House; 2015.
36. Waters F, Collerton D, ffytche DH, et al. Visual hallucinations in the psychosis spectrum and comparative information from neurodegenerative disorders and eye disease. Schizophr Bull. 2014;40(Suppl 4):S233-S245.
37. Gilbert P. The evolution of social mentalities: Compassion and social rank in human psychology. Br J Med Psychol.1998;71(Pt 1):1-22.
38. Burns DD. The Feeling Good Handbook. Plume; 1989.
39. Sheline YI, Barch DM, Price JL, et al. The default mode network and self-referential processes in depression. Proc Natl Acad Sci U S A. 2009;106(6):1942-1947.
40. LeDoux J. Anxious: Using the Brain to Understand and Treat Fear and Anxiety. Penguin Random House; 2015.
41. Langer EJ. The illusion of control. J Pers Soc Psychol. 1975;32(2):311-328.
42. Fenton-O'Creevy M, Nicholson N, Soane E, Willman P. Trading on illusions: Unrealistic perceptions of control and trading performance. J Behav Decis Mak. 2003;16(4):353-376.
43. Gilbert P. Evolution and social anxiety: The role of attraction, social competition, and social hierarchies. Psychiatry.2001;64(3):205-223.
44. Clearer Thinking. (n.d.). The illusion of control: How it shapes decision-making and risk-taking. Retrieved from www.clearerthinking.org
45. Psychological Science. (n.d.). The psychology of "placebo buttons". Retrieved from www.psychologicalscience.org
46. The Decision Lab. (n.d.). The illusion of control: Why we overestimate our influence on events. Retrieved from www.thedecisionlab.com

References

47. Wikipedia. (2023). Illusion of control. Retrieved from https://en.wikipedia.org/wiki/Illusion_of_control
48. Carr, N. (2011). The shallows: What the internet is doing to our brains. W.W. Norton & Company.
49. Chang, A. M., Aeschbach, D., Duffy, J. F., & Czeisler, C. A. (2015). Evening use of light-emitting eReaders negatively affects sleep, circadian timing, and next-morning alertness. Proceedings of the National Academy of Sciences, 112(4), 1232–1237.
50. Elhai, J. D., Levine, J. C., Dvorak, R. D., & Hall, B. J. (2018). Fear of missing out, need for touch, anxiety, and depression among young adults. Computers in Human Behavior, 84, 54-60.
51. Keles, B., McCrae, N., & Grealish, A. (2020). The effects of social media on depression, anxiety, and psychological distress. International Journal of Adolescence and Youth, 25(1), 79-93.
52. Twenge, J. M., Joiner, T. E., Rogers, M. L., & Martin, G. N. (2018). Association between screen time and depression among U.S. adolescents. Preventive Medicine Reports, 12, 271-283.
53. Ferrari, J. R., Roster, C. A., & Crum, K. P. (2018). Decluttering the mind: Examining the relationship between procrastination and clutter across generations. Current Psychology, 37(2), 426-432.
54. Frost, R. O., Steketee, G., & Tolin, D. F. (2012). Excessive acquisition in hoarding disorder. Journal of Anxiety Disorders, 26(5), 525-532.
55. Saxbe, D. E., & Repetti, R. (2010). No place like home: Home tours correlate with daily patterns of mood and cortisol. Personality and Social Psychology Bulletin, 36(1), 71-81.
56. Timpano, K. R., Keough, M. E., & Schmidt, N. B. (2017). Hoarding and sleep quality. Sleep, 40(4), 213-220.
57. Baumeister, R. F., Bratslavsky, E., Muraven, M., & Tice, D. M. (1998). Ego depletion: Is the active self a limited resource? Journal of Personality and Social Psychology, 74(5), 1252–1265.
58. Christakis, N. A., & Fowler, J. H. (2007). The spread of obesity in a large social network over 32 years. New England Journal of Medicine, 357(4), 370-379.
59. Clear, J. (2018). Atomic habits: An easy & proven way to build good habits & break bad ones. Penguin Random House.
60. Duhigg, C. (2012). The power of habit: Why we do what we do in life and business. Random House.
61. Fogg, B. J. (2020). Tiny habits: The small changes that change everything. Houghton Mifflin Harcourt.
62. Neff, K. D. (2011). Self-compassion, self-esteem, and well-being. Social and Personality Psychology Compass, 5(1), 1-12.
63. Brown, K. W., & Ryan, R. M. (2003). The benefits of being present: Mindfulness and its role in psychological well-being. Journal of Personality and Social Psychology, 84(4), 822-848.
64. Duhigg, C. (2012). The power of habit: Why we do what we do in life and business. Random House.
65. Goyal, M., Singh, S., Sibinga, E. M. S., Gould, N. F., Rowland-Seymour, A., Sharma, R., & Haythornthwaite, J. A. (2014). Meditation programs for psychological stress and well-being. JAMA Internal Medicine, 174(3), 357-368.
66. Kabat-Zinn, J. (2013). Full catastrophe living: Using the wisdom of your body and mind to face stress, pain, and illness.Bantam Books.
67. Lally, P., van Jaarsveld, C. H. M., Potts, H. W. W., & Wardle, J. (2010). How are habits formed: Modeling habit formation in the real world. European Journal of Social Psychology, 40(6), 998-1009.
68. Baumeister, R. F., Bratslavsky, E., Finkenauer, C., & Vohs, K. D. (2001). Bad is stronger than good. Review of General Psychology, 5(4), 323–370. https://doi.org/10.1037/1089-2680.5.4.323

69. Doidge, N. (2007). The brain that changes itself: Stories of personal triumph from the frontiers of brain science. Viking.

70. Moruzzi, G., & Magoun, H. W. (1949). Brain stem reticular formation and activation of the EEG. Electroencephalography and Clinical Neurophysiology, 1(4), 455–473. https://doi.org/10.1016/0013-4694(49)90219-9

71. Raz, A., & Buhle, J. (2006). Typologies of attentional networks. Nature Reviews Neuroscience, 7(5), 367–379. https://doi.org/10.1038/nrn1903

72. Mark, G., Wang, Y., & Niiya, M. (2017). Stress and multitasking in everyday college life: An experience sampling study. Proceedings of the SIGCHI Conference on Human Factors in Computing Systems, 891–902. https://doi.org/10.1145/3025453.3025547

73. Ward, A. F., Duke, K., Gneezy, A., & Bos, M. W. (2017). Brain drain: The mere presence of one's own smartphone reduces available cognitive capacity. Journal of the Association for Consumer Research, 2(2), 140–154. https://doi.org/10.1086/691462

74. Frydman, C., & Camerer, C. F. (2016). The psychology and neuroscience of financial decision making. Trends in Cognitive Sciences, 20(9), 661–675. https://doi.org/10.1016/j.tics.2016.07.003

75. McEwen, B. S. (2007). Physiology and neurobiology of stress and adaptation: Central role of the brain. Physiological Reviews, 87(3), 873–904. https://doi.org/10.1152/physrev.00041.2006

76. Rozin, P., & Royzman, E. B. (2001). Negativity bias in psychological research. Review of General Psychology, 5(4), 323–370. https://doi.org/10.1037/1089-2680.5.4.323

77. Soroka, S., Fournier, P., & Nir, L. (2019). Cross-national evidence of a negativity bias in psychophysiological reactions to news. Proceedings of the National Academy of Sciences, 116(38), 18888–18892. https://doi.org/10.1073/pnas.1908369116

78. Alderson-Day B, Fernyhough C. Inner speech: Development, cognitive functions, phenomenology, and neurobiology. Psychol Bull. 2015;141(5):931-965. doi:10.1037/bul0000021

79. Brewer JA, Worhunsky PD, Gray JR, et al. Meditation experience is associated with differences in default mode network activity and connectivity. Proc Natl Acad Sci USA. 2011;108(50):20254-20259. doi:10.1073/pnas.1112029108

80. Buckner RL, Andrews-Hanna JR, Schacter DL. The brain's default network: Anatomy, function, and relevance to disease. Ann N Y Acad Sci. 2008;1124(1):1-38. doi:10.1196/annals.1440.011

81. Corlett PR, Honey GD, Fletcher PC. Prediction error, ketamine and psychosis: An updated model. J Psychopharmacol.2007;21(3):238-258. doi:10.1177/0269881107077716

82. Freeman D, Pugh K, Antley A, et al. Virtual reality study of paranoid thinking in the general population. Br J Psychiatry. 2017;211(5):326-333. doi:10.1192/bjp.bp.117.202419

83. Friston K. The free-energy principle: A unified brain theory? Nat Rev Neurosci. 2010;11(2):127-138. doi:10.1038/nrn2787

84. Garrison KA, Zeffiro TA, Scheinost D, et al. Meditation leads to reduced default mode network activity beyond an active task. Cogn Affect Behav Neurosci. 2015;15(3):712-720. doi:10.3758/s13415-015-0358-3

85. Hayes SC, Strosahl KD, Wilson KG. Acceptance and Commitment Therapy: An Experiential Approach to Behavior Change. Guilford Press; 1999.

86. Nolen-Hoeksema S, Wisco BE, Lyubomirsky S. Rethinking rumination. Perspect Psychol Sci. 2008;3(5):400-424. doi:10.1111/j.1745-6924.2008.00088.x

87. Powers AR, Mathys C, Corlett PR. Pavlovian conditioning-induced hallucinations result from overweighting of perceptual priors. Science. 2017;357(6351):596-600. doi:10.1126/science.aan3458

88. Szechtman H, Woody E. Obsessive-compulsive disorder as a disturbance of security motivation. Psychol Rev.2004;111(1):111-127. doi:10.1037/0033-295x.111.1.111

References

89. Zeidan F, Johnson SK, Diamond BJ, David Z, Goolkasian P. Mindfulness meditation improves cognition: Evidence of brief mental training. Conscious Cogn. 2010;19(2):597-605. doi:10.1016/j.concog.2010.03.014

90. Brewer JA, Worhunsky PD, Gray JR, et al. Meditation experience is associated with differences in default mode network activity and connectivity. Proc Natl Acad Sci USA. 2011;108(50):20254-20259. doi:10.1073/pnas.1112029108

91. Hayes SC, Strosahl KD, Wilson KG. Acceptance and Commitment Therapy: An Experiential Approach to Behavior Change. Guilford Press; 1999.

92. Heppner WL, Kernis MH, Lakey CE, et al. Mindfulness as a means of reducing aggressive behavior: Dispositional and situational evidence. Aggress Behav. 2018;34(5):486-496. doi:10.1002/ab.20258

93. Masuda A, Hayes SC, Sackett CF, Twohig MP. Cognitive defusion and self-relevant negative thoughts: Examining the impact of a ninety-year-old technique. Behav Res Ther. 2004;42(4):477-485. doi:10.1016/j.brat.2003.10.008

94. George MS, Lisanby SH, Avery D, et al. Daily left prefrontal transcranial magnetic stimulation therapy for major depressive disorder: A sham-controlled randomized trial. Arch Gen Psychiatry. 2010;67(5):507-516.

95. Lefaucheur JP, Aleman A, Baeken C, et al. Evidence-based guidelines on the therapeutic use of repetitive transcranial magnetic stimulation (rTMS). Clin Neurophysiol. 2020;131(2):474-528.

96. Berlim MT, Van den Eynde F, Daskalakis ZJ. Clinically meaningful efficacy and acceptability of low-frequency repetitive transcranial magnetic stimulation (rTMS) for treating primary major depression: A meta-analysis of randomized, double-blind and sham-controlled trials. Neuropsychopharmacology. 2013;38(4):543-551.

97. Bath SC, Steer CD, Golding J, Emmett P, Rayman MP. Inadequate iodine status in UK pregnant women and offspring cognitive outcomes. Lancet. 2013;382(9889):331-337.

98. Benton D, Haller J, Fordyce FM. The impact of long-term selenium supplementation on mood in the elderly: A randomized, controlled trial. Biol Psychiatry. 2016;79(1):32-38.

99. Pasco JA, Jacka FN, Williams LJ, Evans-Cleary A, Brennan SL, Berk M. Dietary selenium and major depression: A nested case-control study. J Affect Disord. 2012;141(2-3):141-147.

100. Zimmermann MB. The effects of iodine deficiency in pregnancy and infancy. Paediatr Perinat Epidemiol. 2012;26(suppl 1):108-117.

101. Morris G, Anderson G, Berk M, Maes M. Coenzyme Q10 depletion in medical and neuropsychiatric disorders: potential repercussions and therapeutic implications. Mol Neurobiol. 2013;48(3):883-903.

102. Forester BP, Zuo CS, Ravichandran C, Harper DG, Du F, Kim S, Cohen BM, Renshaw PF. Coenzyme Q10 effects on creatine kinase activity and mood in geriatric bipolar depression. J Geriatr Psychiatry Neurol. 2012;25(1):43-50.

103. Mehrpooya M, Yasrebifar F, Haghighi M, Mohammadi Y, Jahromi GP. The effect of coenzyme Q10 supplementation on oxidative stress and clinical outcomes of depression: a randomized, double-blind, placebo-controlled trial. Brain Behav. 2018;8(9):e01003.

104. Wang Y, Liu XJ, Robitaille L, et al. Plasma vitamin C concentrations and depressive symptoms: a cross-sectional study. J Psychiatr Res. 2013;47(7):928-932.

105. Pullar JM, Carr AC, Vissers MC. The roles of vitamin C in skin health. Nutrients. 2017;9(8):866.

106. Lopresti AL, Hood SD, Drummond PD. A review of lifestyle factors that contribute to important pathways associated with major depression: diet, sleep and exercise. J Affect Disord. 2015;148(1):12-27.

References

107. Grosso G, Pajak A, Marventano S, Castellano S, Galvano F, Bucolo C, Caraci F. Role of omega-3 fatty acids in the treatment of depressive disorders: a comprehensive meta-analysis of randomized clinical trials. PLoS One. 2014;9(5):e96905.

108. Mocking RJ, Harmsen I, Assies J, Koeter MW, Ruhé HG, Schene AH. Meta-analysis and meta-regression of omega-3 polyunsaturated fatty acid supplementation for major depressive disorder. Transl Psychiatry. 2016;6(3):e756.

109. Lin PY, Huang SY, Su KP. A meta-analytic review of polyunsaturated fatty acid compositions in patients with depression. Biol Psychiatry. 2010;68(2):140-147.

110. Kennedy DO. B Vitamins and the Brain: Mechanisms, Dose and Efficacy—A Review. Nutrients. 2016;8(2):68.

111. Rucklidge JJ, Kaplan BJ. Broad-spectrum micronutrient treatment for attention-deficit/ hyperactivity disorder: rationale and evidence to date. CNS Drugs. 2013;27(10):775-785.

112. Sánchez-Villegas A, Henríquez-Sánchez P, Ruiz-Canela M, Lahortiga F, Molero P, Toledo E, Martínez-González MA. A longitudinal analysis of diet quality scores and the risk of incident depression in the SUN Project. BMC Med. 2015;13:197.

113. Rucklidge JJ, Johnstone JM, Kaplan BJ. Nutrition provides the essential foundation for optimizing mental health. Evidence-Based Complement Alternat Med. 2017;2017:9138901.

114. Toussaint L, Worthington EL, Williams DR. Forgiveness and health: Scientific evidence and theories relating forgiveness to better health. New York, NY: Springer; 2016.

115. Wade NG, Hoyt WT, Kidwell JE, Worthington EL. Efficacy of psychotherapeutic interventions to promote forgiveness: A meta-analysis. J Consult Clin Psychol. 2014;82(1):154-170.

116. Akhtar S, Barlow J. Forgiveness therapy for the promotion of mental well-being: a systematic review and meta-analysis. Trauma Violence Abuse. 2018;19(1):107-122.

117. Fredrickson BL, Cohn MA, Coffey KA, Pek J, Finkel SM. Open hearts build lives: Positive emotions, induced through loving-kindness meditation, build consequential personal resources. J Pers Soc Psychol. 2008;95(5):1045-1062.

118. Hall JH, Fincham FD. Self-forgiveness: the stepchild of forgiveness research. J Soc Clin Psychol. 2005;24(5):621-637.

119. Kashdan TB, Rottenberg J. Psychological flexibility as a fundamental aspect of health. Clin Psychol Rev. 2010;30(7):865-878.

120. Hayes SC, Strosahl KD, Wilson KG. Acceptance and commitment therapy: The process and practice of mindful change. 2nd ed. New York, NY: Guilford Press; 2012.

121. Shapiro SL, Carlson LE, Astin JA, Freedman B. Mechanisms of mindfulness. J Clin Psychol. 2006;62(3):373-386.

122. Moncrieff, J., Cooper, R. E., Stockmann, T., Amendola, S., Hengartner, M. P., & Horowitz, M. A. (2022). The serotonin theory of depression: a systematic umbrella review of the evidence. Molecular Psychiatry, 27(7), 1288–1294. https://doi.org/10.1038/s41380-022-01661-0

123. Sathyanarayana Rao, T. S., Asha, M. R., Ramesh, B. N., & Jagannatha Rao, K. S. (2008). Understanding nutrition, depression and mental illnesses. Indian Journal of Psychiatry, 50(2), 77–82. https://doi.org/10.4103/0019-5545.42391

124. Kaplan, B. J., Crawford, S. G., Field, C. J., & Simpson, J. S. (2007). Vitamins, minerals, and mood. Psychological Bulletin, 133(5), 747–760. https://doi.org/10.1037/0033-2909.133.5.747

125. Hengartner, M. P. (2017). Raising awareness for the risks of selective serotonin reuptake inhibitors in depression: a call for balanced reporting. Frontiers in Psychiatry, 8, 188. https://doi.org/10.3389/fpsyt.2017.00188

126. Sarris, J., Logan, A. C., Akbaraly, T. N., et al. (2015). Nutritional medicine as mainstream in psychiatry. The Lancet Psychiatry, 2(3), 271–274. https://doi.org/10.1016/S2215-0366(14)00051-0

References

127. Lacasse, J. R., & Leo, J. (2005). Serotonin and depression: A disconnect between the advertisements and the scientific literature. PLoS Medicine, 2(12), e392. https://doi.org/10.1371/journal.pmed.0020392

128. Almeida, O. P., Flicker, L., Norman, P., et al. (2005). Association of folate and vitamin B12 with depression in later life. British Journal of Psychiatry, 186(6), 475–482. https://doi.org/10.1192/bjp.186.6.475

129. Tarleton, E. K., Littenberg, B., MacLean, C. D., Kennedy, A. G., & Dalessandro, A. M. (2013). Role of magnesium supplementation in the treatment of depression: A randomized clinical trial. Journal of Affective Disorders, 149(1–3), 367–373. https://doi.org/10.1016/j.jad.2013.01.035

130. Whitaker, R. (2010). Anatomy of an Epidemic: Magic Bullets, Psychiatric Drugs, and the Astonishing Rise of Mental Illness in America. Crown Publishing Group.

131. Rucklidge, J. J., Kaplan, B. J., & Mulder, R. T. (2012). Micronutrients in mental health: A review of the evidence. Clinical Psychology Review, 32(6), 881–897. https://doi.org/10.1016/j.cpr.2012.09.004

132. Shin, L. M., Rauch, S. L., & Pitman, R. K. (2006). Amygdala, medial prefrontal cortex, and hippocampal function in PTSD. Annals of the New York Academy of Sciences, 1071(1), 67–79. https://doi.org/10.1196/annals.1364.007

133. van der Kolk, B. A. (2014). The Body Keeps the Score: Brain, Mind, and Body in the Healing of Trauma. Viking.

134. Yehuda, R., McFarlane, A. C., & Shalev, A. Y. (1998). Predicting the development of posttraumatic stress disorder from the acute response to a traumatic event. Biological Psychiatry, 44(12), 1305–1313. https://doi.org/10.1016/S0006-3223(98)00276-5

135. Pagani, M., Di Lorenzo, G., Verardo, A. R., Nicolais, G., Monaco, L., Lauretti, G., ... & Siracusano, A. (2012). Neurobiological correlates of EMDR monitoring – An EEG study. PLOS ONE, 7(9), e45753. https://doi.org/10.1371/journal.pone.0045753

136. Kross, E., & Ayduk, Ö. (2011). Making meaning out of negative experiences by self-distancing. Current Directions in Psychological Science, 20(3), 187–191. https://doi.org/10.1177/0963721411408883

137. Ochsner, K. N., Bunge, S. A., Gross, J. J., & Gabrieli, J. D. E. (2002). Rethinking feelings: An fMRI study of the cognitive regulation of emotion. Journal of Cognitive Neuroscience, 14(8), 1215–1229. https://doi.org/10.1162/089892902760807212

138. Nolen-Hoeksema, S., Wisco, B. E., & Lyubomirsky, S. (2008). Rethinking rumination. Perspectives on Psychological Science, 3(5), 400–424. https://doi.org/10.1111/j.1745-6924.2008.00088.x

139. Lieberman, M. D., Eisenberger, N. I., Crockett, M. J., Tom, S. M., Pfeifer, J. H., & Way, B. M. (2007). Putting feelings into words: Affect labeling disrupts amygdala activity in response to affective stimuli. Psychological Science, 18(5), 421–428. https://doi.org/10.1111/j.1467-9280.2007.01916.x

140. Courtois, C. A., & Ford, J. D. (2009). Treating complex traumatic stress disorders: An evidence-based guide. Guilford Press.

141. Foa, E. B., & Rothbaum, B. O. (1998). Treating the trauma of rape: Cognitive-behavioral therapy for PTSD. Guilford Press.

142. Herman, J. L. (1992). Trauma and recovery: The aftermath of violence—from domestic abuse to political terror. Basic Books.

143. Neimeyer, R. A. (2000). Searching for the meaning of meaning: Grief therapy and the process of reconstruction. Death Studies, 24(6), 541–558. https://doi.org/10.1080/07481180050121480

144. Thompson, R. W., Arnkoff, D. B., & Glass, C. R. (2021). Conceptualizing mindfulness and acceptance as components of psychological resilience to trauma. Trauma, Violence, & Abuse, 22(1), 78–92. https://doi.org/10.1177/1524838018821304

145.Courtois, C. A., & Ford, J. D. (2009). Treating complex traumatic stress disorders: An evidence-based guide. Guilford Press.

146.Foa, E. B., & Rothbaum, B. O. (1998). Treating the trauma of rape: Cognitive-behavioral therapy for PTSD. Guilford Press.

147.Herman, J. L. (1992). Trauma and recovery: The aftermath of violence—from domestic abuse to political terror. Basic Books.

148.Neimeyer, R. A. (2000). Searching for the meaning of meaning: Grief therapy and the process of reconstruction. Death Studies, 24(6), 541–558. https://doi.org/10.1080/07481180050121480

149.Thompson, R. W., Arnkoff, D. B., & Glass, C. R. (2021). Conceptualizing mindfulness and acceptance as components of psychological resilience to trauma. Trauma, Violence, & Abuse, 22(1), 78–92. https://doi.org/10.1177/1524838018821304

150.Beck, J. S. (2011). Cognitive behavior therapy: Basics and beyond (2nd ed.). New York: Guilford Press.

151.Cuijpers, P., Berking, M., Andersson, G., Quigley, L., Kleiboer, A., & Dobson, K. S. (2013). A meta-analysis of cognitive-behavioral therapy for adult depression, alone and in comparison with other treatments. The Canadian Journal of Psychiatry, 58(7), 376–385. https://doi.org/10.1177/070674371305800700

152.Kazantzis, N., Whittington, C., & Dattilio, F. (2018). Meta-analysis of homework effects in cognitive and behavioral therapy: A replication and extension. Clinical Psychology: Science and Practice, 17(2), 144–156.

153.Segal, Z. V., Williams, J. M. G., & Teasdale, J. D. (2013). Mindfulness-based cognitive therapy for depression (2nd ed.). New York: Guilford Press.

154.Abbey, G., Thompson, S. B., Hickish, T., & Heathcote, D. (2015). A meta-analysis of prevalence rates and moderating factors for cancer-related post-traumatic stress disorder. Psycho-Oncology, 24(4), 371–381. https://doi.org/10.1002/pon.3654

155.Levine, P. A. (2008). Healing trauma: A pioneering program for restoring the wisdom of your body. Boulder, CO: Sounds True.

156.Shapiro, F. (2018). Eye Movement Desensitization and Reprocessing (EMDR) therapy: Basic principles, protocols, and procedures (3rd ed.). New York: Guilford Press.

157.Van der Kolk, B. A. (2015). The body keeps the score: Brain, mind, and body in the healing of trauma. New York: Viking.

158.American Psychiatric Association. Diagnostic and Statistical Manual of Mental Disorders. 5th ed. American Psychiatric Publishing; 2022.

159.Craske MG, Stein MB, Eley TC, et al. Anxiety disorders. Nat Rev Dis Primers. 2017;3:17024. doi:10.1038/nrdp.2017.24

160.Roy-Byrne PP, Craske MG, Stein MB. Panic disorder. Lancet. 2006;368(9540):1023-1032. doi:10.1016/S0140-6736(06)69418-X

161.Stein MB, Stein DJ. Social anxiety disorder. Lancet. 2008;371(9618):1115-1125. doi:10.1016/S0140-6736(08)60488-2

162.Hettema JM, Neale MC, Kendler KS. A review and meta-analysis of the genetic epidemiology of anxiety disorders. Am J Psychiatry. 2001;158(10):1568-1578. doi:10.1176/appi.ajp.158.10.1568

163.Shin LM, Liberzon I. The neurocircuitry of fear, stress, and anxiety disorders. Neuropsychopharmacology. 2010;35(1):169-191. doi:10.1038/npp.2009.83

164.Arnsten AFT. Stress signalling pathways that impair prefrontal cortex structure and function. Nat Rev Neurosci. 2009;10(6):410-422. doi:10.1038/nrn2648

165.McEwen BS. Physiology and neurobiology of stress and adaptation: central role of the brain. Physiol Rev. 2007;87(3):873-904. doi:10.1152/physrev.00041.2006

References

166. Beck AT, Clark DA. An information processing model of anxiety: automatic and strategic processes. Behav Res Ther. 1997;35(1):49-58. doi:10.1016/S0005-7967(96)00069-1

167. Glaser R, Kiecolt-Glaser JK. Stress-induced immune dysfunction: implications for health. Nat Rev Immunol. 2005;5(3):243-251. doi:10.1038/nri1571

168. Tang YY, Hölzel BK, Posner MI. The neuroscience of mindfulness meditation. Nat Rev Neurosci. 2015;16(4):213-225. doi:10.1038/nrn3916

169. Jacka FN, O'Neil A, Opie R, et al. A randomised controlled trial of dietary improvement for adults with major depression (the 'SMILES' trial). BMC Med. 2017;15(1):23. doi:10.1186/s12916-017-0791-y

170. Lassale C, Batty GD, Baghdadli A, et al. Healthy dietary indices and risk of depressive outcomes: a systematic review and meta-analysis of observational studies. Mol Psychiatry. 2019;24(7):965-986. doi:10.1038/s41380-018-0237-8

171. Marx W, Moseley G, Berk M, Jacka F, O'Neil A, Itsiopoulos C. Nutritional psychiatry: the present state of the evidence. Proc Nutr Soc. 2021;80(4):403-412. doi:10.1017/S0029665121000016

172. Beck AT. Cognitive Therapy and the Emotional Disorders. International Universities Press; 1976.

173. Shin LM, Liberzon I. The neurocircuitry of fear, stress, and anxiety disorders. Neuropsychopharmacology.2010;35(1):169-191. doi:10.1038/npp.2009.83

174. Clark DA, Beck AT. Cognitive Therapy of Anxiety Disorders: Science and Practice. Guilford Press; 2010.

175. Nolen-Hoeksema S, Wisco BE, Lyubomirsky S. Rethinking rumination. Perspect Psychol Sci. 2008;3(5):400-424. doi:10.1111/j.1745-6924.2008.00088.x

176. Watkins ER. Constructive and unconstructive repetitive thought. Psychol Bull. 2008;134(2):163-206. doi:10.1037/0033-2909.134.2.163

177. Shin LM, Liberzon I. The neurocircuitry of fear, stress, and anxiety disorders. Neuropsychopharmacology.2010;35(1):169-191. doi:10.1038/npp.2009.83

178. Whitmer AJ, Gotlib IH. Switching and backward inhibition in major depressive disorder: the role of rumination. J Abnorm Psychol. 2012;121(3):570-578. doi:10.1037/a0027474

179. Beck AT. Cognitive Therapy and the Emotional Disorders. International Universities Press; 1976.

180. Shin LM, Rauch SL, Pitman RK. Amygdala, medial prefrontal cortex, and hippocampal function in PTSD. Ann N Y Acad Sci. 2006;1071:67-79. doi:10.1196/annals.1364.007

181. Rauch SL, Shin LM, Phelps EA. Neurocircuitry models of posttraumatic stress disorder and extinction: Human neuroimaging research past, present, and future. Biol Psychiatry. 2006;60(4):376-382. doi:10.1016/j.biopsych.2006.06.004

182. Van der Kolk BA. The Body Keeps the Score: Brain, Mind, and Body in the Healing of Trauma. Viking; 2014.

183. Shapiro F. Eye Movement Desensitization and Reprocessing (EMDR) Therapy: Basic Principles, Protocols, and Procedures. 3rd ed. Guilford Press; 2017.

184. Thayer, J. F., Åhs, F., Fredrikson, M., Sollers, J. J., & Wager, T. D. (2012). A meta-analysis of heart rate variability and neuroimaging studies: Implications for heart rate variability as a marker of stress and health. Neuroscience & Biobehavioral Reviews, 36(2), 747–756. https://doi.org/10.1016/j.neubiorev.2011.11.009

185. Pitman, R. K., Rasmusson, A. M., Koenen, K. C., Shin, L. M., Orr, S. P., Gilbertson, M. W., … Liberzon, I. (2012). Biological studies of post-traumatic stress disorder. Nature Reviews Neuroscience, 13(11), 769–787. https://doi.org/10.1038/nrn3339

186. Shin, L. M., & Liberzon, I. (2010). The neurocircuitry of fear, stress, and anxiety disorders. Neuropsychopharmacology, 35(1), 169–191. https://doi.org/10.1038/npp.2009.83

187. Yehuda, R. (2002). Post-traumatic stress disorder. New England Journal of Medicine, 346(2), 108–114. https://doi.org/10.1056/NEJMra012941

References

188. McCorry, L. K. (2007). Physiology of the autonomic nervous system. American Journal of Pharmaceutical Education, 71(4), 78. https://doi.org/10.5688/aj710478

189. Williamson, A., & Hoggart, B. (2005). Pain: A review of three commonly used pain rating scales. Journal of Clinical Nursing, 14(7), 798–804. https://doi.org/10.1111/j.1365-2702.2005.01121.x

190. https://advancedsofttissuerelease.com/biopsycho-therapy-bpt-psychotherapy-course/

www.ingramcontent.com/pod-product-compliance
Lightning Source LLC
Chambersburg PA
CBHW052020030426
42335CB00026B/3220